MILADY STANDARD ESTHETICS
FUNDAMENTALS

Step-by-Step Procedures

MILADY STANDARD ESTHETICS FUNDAMENTALS

Step-by-Step Procedures

Joel Gerson

Contributors:

Janet D'Angelo

Sallie Deitz

Shelley Lotz

Editorial Contributor:

Letha Barnes

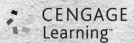

CENGAGE
Learning™

Australia • Brazil • Japan • Korea • Mexico • Singapore • Spain • United Kingdom • United States

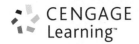
CENGAGE Learning™

Milady Standard Esthetics: Fundamentals Step-by-Step Procedures, Eleventh Edition

Author (s): Joel Gerson, Janet D'Angelo, Sallie Deitz, Shelley Lotz, and Letha Barnes

Vice President, Milady & Learning Solutions Strategy, Professional: Dawn Gerrain

Director of Content & Business Development, Milady: Sandra Bruce

Associate Acquisitions Editor: Philip I. Mandl

Senior Product Manager: Jessica Mahoney

Editorial Assistant: Sarah Prediletto

Director, Marketing & Training: Gerard McAvey

Marketing Manager: Matthew McGuire

Senior Production Director: Wendy A. Troeger

Production Manager: Sherondra Thedford

Senior Content Project Manager: Nina Tucciarelli

Senior Art Director: Benj Gleeksman

For product information and technology assistance, contact us at
Cengage Learning Customer & Sales Support, 1-800-354-9706
For permission to use material from this text or product,
submit all requests online at **www.cengage.com/permissions**.
Further permissions questions can be e-mailed to
permissionrequest@cengage.com.

Library of Congress Control Number: 2011943910

ISBN-13: 978-1-1113-0709-7
ISBN-10: 1-1113-0709-1

Milady
5 Maxwell Drive
Clifton Park, NY 12065-2919
USA

Cengage Learning is a leading provider of customized learning solutions with office locations around the globe, including Singapore, the United Kingdom, Australia, Mexico, Brazil, and Japan. Locate your local office at: **international. cengage.com/region**

Cengage Learning products are represented in Canada by Nelson Education, Ltd.

For your lifelong learning solutions, visit **milady.cengage.com**

Purchase any of our products at your local college store or at our preferred online store **www.cengagebrain.com**

Visit our corporate website at **cengage.com**.

Notice to the Reader

Publisher does not warrant or guarantee any of the products described herein or perform any independent analysis in connection with any of the product information contained herein. Publisher does not assume, and expressly disclaims, any obligation to obtain and include information other than that provided to it by the manufacturer. The reader is expressly warned to consider and adopt all safety precautions that might be indicated by the activities described herein and to avoid all potential hazards. By following the instructions contained herein, the reader willingly assumes all risks in connection with such instructions. The publisher makes no representations or warranties of any kind, including but not limited to, the warranties of fitness for particular purpose or merchantability, nor are any such representations implied with respect to the material set forth herein, and the publisher takes no responsibility with respect to such material. The publisher shall not be liable for any special, consequential, or exemplary damages resulting, in whole or part, from the readers' use of, or reliance upon, this material.

Printed in United States of America
1 2 3 4 5 XX 16 15 14 13 12

Table of Contents

How to Use This Workbook

Congratulations on purchasing this step-by-step procedures book, a companion to your Milady Standard Esthetics: Fundamentals, 11th Edition, textbook. You can use this book in conjunction with your textbook, or on its own to brush up on key procedures. Each step is clearly explained and is accompanied throughout by full color photos.

Performance Rubrics

At the end of each procedure, you'll find a list of rubrics, or ways to note and comment on your performance for each of the key tasks. Rubrics are used in education for organizing and interpreting data gathered from observations of student performance. Rubrics are specifically developed scoring documents used to differentiate between levels of development in a specific skill performance or behavior. You can use rubrics to evaluate yourself, other estheticians, and other students. As an instructor, you can use rubrics to evaluate you own students.

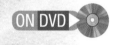

What's on the DVD?

To assist you in really learning each and every step, we've noted which procedures can be found on the companion DVD set, *Milady Standard Esthetics: Fundamentals*. If you already own these DVDs, or know that your school owns them, we encourage you to watch the procedure in video to strengthen your understanding of that particular procedure.

Other Companion Products

Other products in this same product line that may be of interest to you, the practicing or future esthetician:

Milady Standard Esthetics: Fundamentals, 11th Edition
Joel Gerson
ISBN-13: 9781111306892
ISBN-10: 1111306893
© 2013

Milady Standard Esthetics: Fundamentals, DVD Series Milady
ISBN-13: 9781435402812
ISBN-10:1435402812
© 2013

Milady Standard Esthetics: Fundamentals, Student Workbook Milady
ISBN-13: 9781111306915
ISBN-10: 1111306915
© 2013

Milady Standard Esthetics: Fundamentals Online Licensing Preparation, Slimline
Milady
ISBN-13: 9781111307042
ISBN-10:1111307040
© 2013

Milady Standard Esthetics: Fundamentals, Exam Review
Milady
ISBN-13: 9781111306922
ISBN-10: 1111306923
© 2013

Milady Standard Esthetics: Fundamentals, Student CD ROM
Milady
ISBN-13: 9781111306946
ISBN-10: 111130694Xw
© 2013

Milady Standard Esthetics: Fundamentals, Spanish Version
Milady
ISBN-13: 9781111306991
ISBN-10: 1111306990
© 2013

Milady Standard Esthetics: Fundamentals, Exam Review, Spanish Version
Milady
ISBN-13: 9781111306939
ISBN-10: 1111306931
© 2013

Milady Standard Esthetics: Fundamentals, Student Workbook, Spanish Version
Milady
ISBN-13: 9781111306960
ISBN-10: 1111306966
© 2013

Milady's Standard Esthetics: Advanced
Milady
ISBN-13: 978428319752
ISBN-10: 1428319751
© 2013

For more products serving practicing and future estheticians, please visit
www.milady.cengage.com

Step-by-Step Procedures

PROCEDURE 5-1

Disinfecting Nonelectrical Tools and Implements

Nonelectrical tools and implements include items such as comedone extractors, microdermabrasion hand pieces, galvanic accessories, makeup brushes, and tweezers.

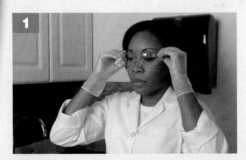

1 It is important to wear safety glasses and gloves while disinfecting nonelectrical tools and implements to protect your eyes from unintentional splashes of disinfectant and to prevent possible contamination of the implements by your hands and to protect your hands from the powerful chemicals in the disinfectant solution.

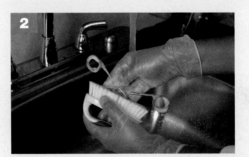

2 Rinse all implements with warm running water, and then thoroughly clean them with soap, a nail brush, and warm water. Brush grooved items, if necessary, and open hinged implements to scrub the revealed area.

© Milady, a part of Cengage Learning. Photography by Dino Petrocelli.

2

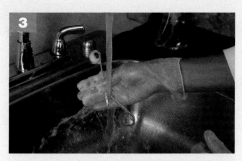

3 Rinse away all traces of soap with warm running water. The presence of soap in most disinfectants will cause them to become inactive. Soap is most easily rinsed off in warm, not hot, water. Hotter water is not more effective. Dry implements thoroughly with a clean or disposable towel, or allow them to air dry on a clean towel. Your implements are now properly cleaned and ready to be disinfected.

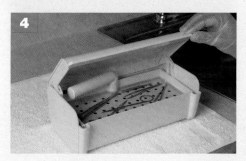

4 It is extremely important that your implements be completely clean before you place them in the disinfectant solution. If implements are not clean, your disinfectant may become contaminated and ineffective. Immerse cleaned implements in an appropriate disinfection container holding an EPA-registered disinfectant for the required time (at least 10 minutes or according to the manufacturer's instructions). Remember to open hinged implements before immersing them in the disinfectant. If the disinfection solution is visibly dirty, or if the solution has been contaminated, it must be replaced.

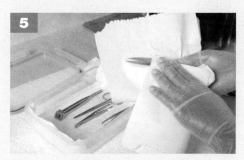

5 After the required disinfection time has passed, remove tools and implements from the disinfection solution with tongs or gloved hands, rinse the tools and implements well in warm running water, and pat them dry.

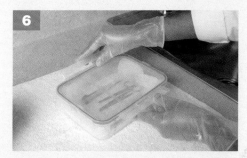

6 Store disinfected tools and implements in a clean, covered container until needed.

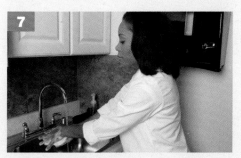

7 Remove gloves and thoroughly wash your hands with warm running water and liquid soap. Rinse and dry hands with a clean fabric or disposable towel.

Rubrics are used in education for organizing and interpreting data gathered from observations of student performance. It is a clearly developed scoring document used to differentiate between levels of development in a specific skill performance or behavior. A rubric is provided in this study guide as a self-assessment tool to aid you in your behavior development.

Rate your performance according to the following scale:

1 **Development Opportunity:** There is little or no evidence of competency; assistance is needed; performance includes multiple errors.

2 **Fundamental:** There is beginning evidence of competency; task is completed alone; performance includes few errors.

3 **Competent:** There is detailed and consistent evidence of competency; task is completed alone; performance includes rare errors.

4 **Strength:** There is detailed evidence of highly creative, inventive, mature presence of competency.

Space is provided for comments to assist you in improving your performance and achieving a higher rating.

Disinfecting Nonelectrical Tools and Implements Assessment

PERFORMANCE ASSESSED	1	2	3	4	IMPROVEMENT PLAN
1. Wore safety glasses and gloves.					
2. Rinsed implements with warm water.					
3. Washed implements with soap and warm water.					
4. Rinsed and dried implements.					
5. Immersed clean implements in disinfectant.					
6. Removed implements with tongs or gloved hands.					
7. Rinsed implements with warm water and patted dry.					
8. Stored disinfected implements properly.					
9. Removed gloves and washed hands.					
10. Rinsed and dried hands.					

Notes

Aseptic Procedure

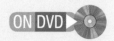ON DVD ▶ ⊙

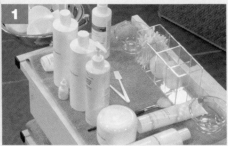

© Milady, a part of Cengage Learning.
Photography by Larry Hamill.

1 Before beginning any treatment, wash your hands using proper decontamination methods.

2 Lay out on a clean towel all implements that you will use during the treatment, such as cotton, swabs, sponges, and so forth.

3 To prevent airborne contact, cover with another clean towel until you are ready to start the treatment. By prearranging these utensils, you will be less likely to need to open a container to get more supplies. This not only prevents cross-contamination but is also more efficient.

4 Once you have begun a treatment, never open any package or container or touch a product without a spatula or tongs. Touching any object with gloved hands that have touched the client will contaminate that object. Any object touched during treatment must be discarded, disinfected, or autoclaved.

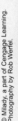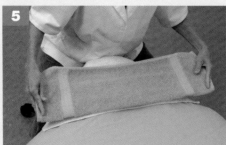

© Milady, a part of Cengage Learning.
Photography by Rob Werfel.

5 Use clean towels, sheets, headband or plastic cap, and gown for each client.

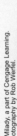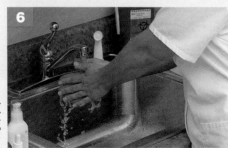

© Milady, a part of Cengage Learning.
Photography by Rob Werfel.

6 Wash your hands after touching a client's hair.

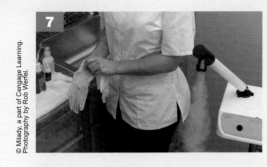

7 Put on gloves at the beginning of every treatment and wear them throughout the treatment. This is especially important during and after extraction, waxing, and the performance of microdermabrasion, skin peels, or electrolysis.

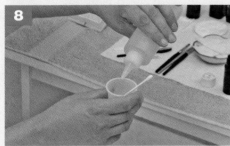

8 Remove creams and products from containers using pumps, squeeze bottles with dispenser caps, or disinfected spatulas. It is best to remove products before the treatment and place them in small disposable cups. This way, you will not have to touch bottles or jars with soiled gloved hands. Spatulas should be disinfected or discarded after each use.

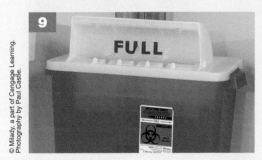

9 After completing the treatment, fold linens in toward their center, then place them in a covered laundry receptacle. Throw away disposable items in a closed trash container. Place sharps in a sharps box. Disinfect or sterilize all items to be reused. Discard any unused product that has been removed from its container.

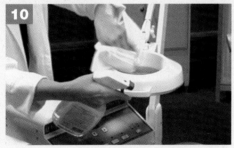

10 Wipe down all surfaces touched during treatment with a disinfectant before the next client is seated.

Rubrics are used in education for organizing and interpreting data gathered from observations of student performance. It is a clearly developed scoring document used to differentiate between levels of development in a specific skill performance or behavior. A rubric is provided in this study guide as a self-assessment tool to aid you in your behavior development.

Rate your performance according to the following scale:

1 **Development Opportunity:** There is little or no evidence of competency; assistance is needed; performance includes multiple errors.

2 **Fundamental:** There is beginning evidence of competency; task is completed alone; performance includes few errors.

3 **Competent:** There is detailed and consistent evidence of competency; task is completed alone; performance includes rare errors.

4 **Strength:** There is detailed evidence of highly creative, inventive, mature presence of competency.

Space is provided for comments to assist you in improving your performance and achieving a higher rating.

Asceptic Procedure Assessment

PERFORMANCE ASSESSED	1	2	3	4	IMPROVEMENT PLAN
1. Washed hands.					
2. Laid out needed implements on clean towel.					
3. Covered implements with another clean towel.					
4. Used spatula or tongs to open packages and handle products.					
5. Used clean towels, sheets, headbands or plastic caps, and gowns.					
6. Washed hands after touching the client.					
7. Wore gloves during entire treatment.					
8. Removed creams and products using pumps, squeeze bottles, or disinfected spatulas.					
9. Spatulas were clean and disinfected or discarded after each use.					
10. Folded used linens in toward center and placed in laundry receptacle.					
11. Discarded disposable items in closed trash container.					
12. Placed sharps in a sharp box.					
13. Disinfected all reusable items.					
14. Discarded all unused product that had been removed from container.					
15. Wiped down all touched surfaces with disinfectant.					

Notes

Proper Hand Washing

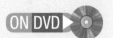

Hand washing is one of the most important procedures in your infection control efforts and is required in every state before any service.

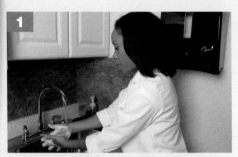

1 Turn on the warm water, wet your hands, and then pump soap from a pump container onto the palm of your hand. Rub your hands together, all over and vigorously, until a lather forms. Continue for a minimum of 20 seconds.

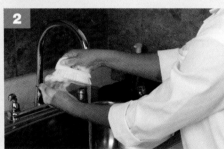

2 Choose a clean, disinfected nail brush. Wet the nail brush, pump soap on it, and brush your nails horizontally back and forth under the free edges. Change the direction of the brush to vertical and move the brush up and down along the nail folds of the fingernails. The process for brushing both hands should take about 60 seconds to finish. Rinse hands in running warm water.

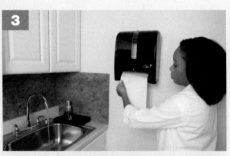

3 Use a clean cloth or paper towel, according to the salon policies, for drying your hands.

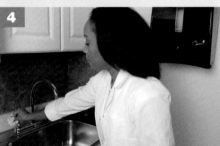

4 After drying your hands, turn off the water with the towel and dispose of the towel.

5-2

Rubrics are used in education for organizing and interpreting data gathered from observations of student performance. It is a clearly developed scoring document used to differentiate between levels of development in a specific skill performance or behavior. A rubric is provided in this study guide as a self-assessment tool to aid you in your behavior development.

Rate your performance according to the following scale:

1 **Development Opportunity:** There is little or no evidence of competency; assistance is needed; performance includes multiple errors.

2 **Fundamental:** There is beginning evidence of competency; task is completed alone; performance includes few errors.

3 **Competent:** There is detailed and consistent evidence of competency; task is completed alone; performance includes rare errors.

4 **Strength:** There is detailed evidence of highly creative, inventive, mature presence of competency.

Space is provided for comments to assist you in improving your performance and achieving a higher rating.

Proper Hand Washing Assessment

PERFORMANCE ASSESSED	1	2	3	4	IMPROVEMENT PLAN
1. Washed hands in soap and water for 20 seconds.					
2. Brushed nails horizontally and vertically with a clean, disinfected nail brush.					
3. Changed directions and brushed for about 60 seconds.					
4. Dried hands with a clean cloth or paper towel.					
5. Turned off water with towel.					
6. Disposed of towel.					

Supplies
- EPA-registered disinfectant
- Hand sanitizer
- Antibacterial soap
- Covered trash container
- Bowl
- Spatula
- Hand towels
- Headband
- Clean linens
- Bolster

Single-use Items
- Gloves
- Cotton pads (4" x 4" for cleansing)
- Cotton rounds
- Cotton swabs
- Plastic bag
- Paper towels
- Tissues

Products
- Eye makeup remover or cleanser
- Facial cleanser
- Toner
- Moisturizer

ON DVD ▶

Performing a Skin Analysis: Step by Step

Preparation

- **Perform** **14-1** PROCEDURE **Pre-Service Procedure** PAGE 16

Procedure

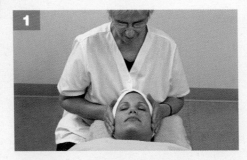

1 Look briefly at your client's skin with your naked eye or a magnifying light. You cannot do an accurate analysis if your client is wearing makeup.

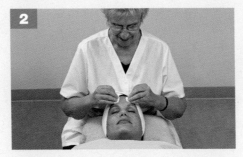

2 Cleanse the skin (a client's normal state of dryness or oiliness may not be as visible immediately after cleansing).

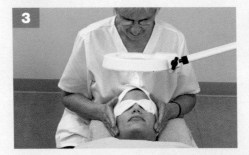

3 Use a magnifying light to examine the skin more thoroughly. Cover the eyes with eye pads. (In addition to the magnifying light, a Wood's lamp can be used here.)

© Milady, a part of Cengage Learning. Photography by Rob Werfel.

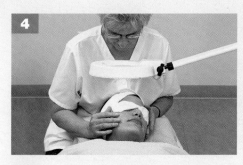

4 Look closely at the client's skin type, the conditions present, and the appearance; also *touch* the skin with the fingertips to feel its texture.

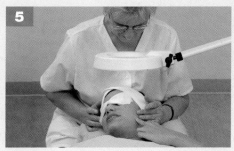

5 Listen: Conduct a brief *consultation* while continuing to analyze with the magnifying lamp.

The four components of skin analysis are *look, feel, ask,* and *listen*.

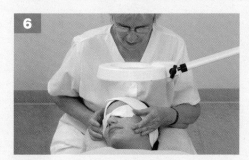

6 Ask questions relating to the skin's appearance and the client's personal health or lifestyle. Discuss what you see with the client; also recommend products and a home-care routine.

7 Reapply a toner and moisturizer or sunscreen to balance and protect the skin.

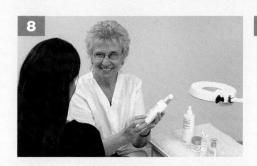

8 Choose products for treatment and home-care.

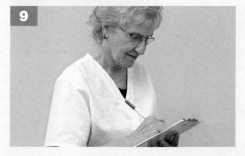

9 Record the information on the client chart at the appropriate time—usually after the treatment is completed.

Post-Service

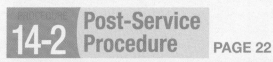

• **Complete** **PROCEDURE** **14-2** **Post-Service Procedure** PAGE 22

© Milady, a part of Cengage Learning. Photography by Rob Werfel.

Rubrics are used in education for organizing and interpreting data gathered from observations of student performance. It is a clearly developed scoring document used to differentiate between levels of development in a specific skill performance or behavior. Rubrics are provided in this supplement for use as either a self-assessment tool to aid the student in behavior development or as an educator assessment tool to determine competence. Space is provided to record steps needed for further growth and improvement.

Performance is evaluated according to the following scale:

1 **Development Opportunity:** There is little or no evidence of competency; assistance is needed; performance includes multiple errors.

2 **Fundamental:** There is beginning evidence of competency; task is completed alone; performance includes few errors.

3 **Competent:** There is detailed and consistent evidence of competency; task is completed alone; performance includes rare errors.

4 **Strength:** There is detailed evidence of highly creative, inventive, mature presence of competency.

Space is provided for comments to assist you in improving your performance and achieving a higher rating.

Performing a Skin Analysis: Step by Step Assessment

PERFORMANCE ASSESSED	1	2	3	4	IMPROVEMENT PLAN
Preparation					
1. Completed standard pre-service procedure.					
Procedure					
1. Observed client's skin with naked eye.					
2. Cleansed client's skin.					
3. Covered eyes with eye pads.					
4. Examined client's skin with magnifying light.					
5. Examined client's skin texture through touch.					
6. Asked questions relating to skin appearance and client's health.					
7. Discussed observations with client.					
8. Recommended home-care products.					
9. Recommended home-care routine.					
10. Reapplied toner and moisturizer or sunscreen to balance and protect skin.					
11. Chose products for treatment and home-care.					
12. Recorded information on client chart after treatment.					
Post-Service					
1. Completed standard post-service procedure, cleanup, and disinfection procedures.					

Notes

PROCEDURE
14-1

Pre-Service Procedure

A. Preparing the Facial Room

Check your room supply of linens (towels and sheets) and replenish as needed. For the first appointment of the day, preheat your towel warmer, towels, wax heater, steamer, and any other equipment as needed.

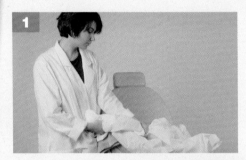

1 Change the bed or treatment chair linens.

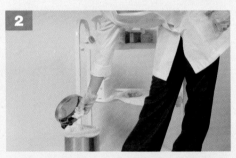

2 Throw away any disposables used during the previous service.

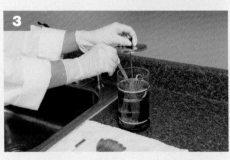

3 Clean and disinfect any used brushes or implements such as mask brushes, comedo extractors, tweezers, machine attachments, and electrodes. See Procedure 5–1, Disinfecting Nonelectrical Tools and Implements on page 2, to clean and disinfect implements properly.

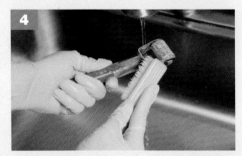

4 Clean and disinfect any machine parts used during the previous service.

Service Tip

Before servicing a client, take a moment to sit on your facial chair and take a good look around. Based on what you see, hear, and feel, ask yourself this question: What kind of an experience will my client have while she is here?

Answering the following questions will enable you to provide your client with a positive experience:

- Is my room clean and organized or cluttered and messy?
- Will the music and the temperature be comfortable for the client?
- Am I wearing too much perfume/ cologne? Am I carrying an unpleasant food or tobacco odor? Is my breath pleasant-smelling?
- When I look at myself in the mirror, do I see the professional I want to be? Does my personal grooming—my hair, makeup, and clothing—look professional?
- Do I look as if I am happy and enjoying my work?
- Is there some problem bothering me today that is affecting my ability to concentrate on the needs of my client?

Remember the old adage: You only get one chance to make a good first impression. Stack the odds in your favor!

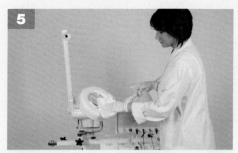

5 Clean and disinfect counters and magnifying lamp or lens.

6 Check the water level on the steamer/vaporizer as needed.

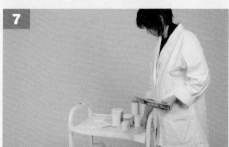

7 Replace any disposable implements you may need such as gloves, sheet cotton, gauze squares, sponges for cleansing and makeup, disposable makeup applicators (mascara wands, lip brushes, other brushes), spatulas and tongue-depressor wax applicators, cotton swabs, facial tissue, and wax strips.

8 Prepare to greet your next client.

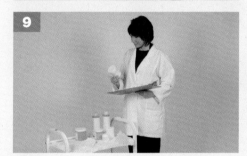

9 Review your client schedule for the day and decide which products you are likely to need for each service. Make sure you have enough of all the products you will be using that day. You may have to retrieve additional product from the dispensary. This is also a good time to refresh your mind about each repeat client you will be seeing that day and his or her individual concerns.

10 Place supplies on a clean towel or cloth in the order to be used, lined up neatly, and cover with another towel until you are ready to use them.

11 Your room should be ready to go from the previous night's thorough cleaning. (See "At the End of the Day" in Procedure 14–2, Post-Service Procedure.)

B. Preparing for the Client

12 Retrieve the client's intake form or service record card and review it. If the appointment is for a new client, let the receptionist know that the client will need an intake form.

13 Organize yourself by taking care of your personal needs before the client arrives—use the restroom, get a drink of water, return a personal call—so that when your client arrives, you can place your full attention on her needs.

14 Turn off cell phone, pager, or PDA. Be sure that you eliminate anything that can distract you from your client while she is in the salon.

15 Take a moment to clear your head of all your personal concerns and issues. Take a couple of deep breaths and remind yourself that you are committed to providing your clients with fantastic service and your full attention.

16 Wash your hands using Procedure 5–3, Proper Hand Washing on page 10, before going to greet your client.

14-1 Pre-Service Procedure (continued)

C. Greet Client

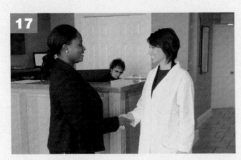

17 Greet your client in the reception area with a warm smile and in a professional manner. Introduce yourself if you've never met, and shake hands. The handshake is the first acceptance by the client of your touch, so be sure your handshake is firm and sincere. If the client is new, ask her for the intake form she filled out in the reception area.

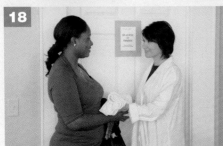

18 Escort the client to the changing area for her to change into a smock or robe. Make sure you tell her where to securely place her personal items. If you do not have a changing room or lockers, she will need to change in the treatment room.

19 Ask the client to remove all jewelry and put in a safe place because you do not want to stop the service for her to remove the jewelry later.

20 Invite her to take a seat in the treatment chair or to lie down on the treatment table.

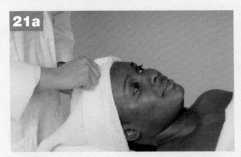

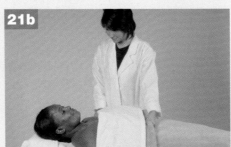

21 Drape the client properly and either place her hair in a protective cap or use a headband and towels to drape her hair properly. Give her a blanket and make sure she is comfortable before beginning the service. Remember, the client is not just a facial or another service, but a person you want to build a relationship with. By first showing clients respect, you will begin to gain their trust in you as a professional. Openness, honesty, and sincerity are always the most successful approach in winning clients' trust, respect, and, ultimately, their loyalty.

22 Perform a consultation before beginning the service. If you are servicing a returning client, ask how her skin has been since her last treatment. If the client is new, discuss the information on the intake form, and ask any questions you have regarding her skin or any conditions listed on the form. Determine a course of action for the treatment, and briefly explain your plan to the client.

Rubrics are used in education for organizing and interpreting data gathered from observations of student performance. It is a clearly developed scoring document used to differentiate between levels of development in a specific skill performance or behavior. Rubrics are provided in this supplement for use as either a self-assessment tool to aid the student in behavior development or as an educator assessment tool to determine competence. Space is provided to record steps needed for further growth and improvement.

Performance is evaluated according to the following scale:

1 Development Opportunity: There is little or no evidence of competency; assistance is needed; performance includes multiple errors.

2 Fundamental: There is beginning evidence of competency; task is completed alone; performance includes few errors.

3 Competent: There is detailed and consistent evidence of competency; task is completed alone; performance includes rare errors.

4 Strength: There is detailed evidence of highly creative, inventive, mature presence of competency.

Space is provided for comments to assist you in improving your performance and achieving a higher rating.

Check your room supply of linens (towels and sheets) and replenish as needed. For the first appointment of the day, preheat your towel warmer, towels, wax heater, steamer, and any other equipment needed.

Pre-Service Procedure Assessment

PERFORMANCE ASSESSED	1	2	3	4	IMPROVEMENT PLAN
Preparing the Facial Room					
1. Changed the bed or treatment chair linens.					
2. Threw away any disposables used during the previous service.					
3. Cleaned and disinfected any used brushes or implements.					
4. Cleaned and disinfected any machine parts used during the previous service.					
5. Cleaned and disinfected counters and magnifying lamp or lens.					
6. Checked water level on vaporizer as needed.					
7. Replaced any disposable implements needed (gloves, sheet cotton, gauze, etc.).					
8. Prepared to greet next client.					
9. Reviewed client schedule and determined needed products.					
10. Placed supplies on a clean towel or cloth in the order to be used and covered with another towel.					
Preparing for the Client					
1. Retrieved client's intake form.					
2. Took care of personal needs before client arrived (restroom, drink of water, returned calls, etc.).					

PERFORMANCE ASSESSED	1	2	3	4	IMPROVEMENT PLAN
3. Turned off cell phone, pager or PDA; eliminated all distractions.					
4. Washed hands according to procedure.					
Greet Client					
1. Greeted client in reception area with a warm smile in a professional manner.					
2. If never met, introduced self.					
3. Shook hands with client.					
4. If new client, requested intake form.					
5. Escorted client to changing area.					
6. Informed client where to place personal items.					
7. Asked client to remove all jewelry and put in safe place.					
8. Invited client to take a seat in treatment chair or lie down on treatment table.					
9. Draped client properly.					
10. Placed hair in protective cap or used headband and towels.					
11. Provided blanket and ensured client comfort.					
12. Performed client consultation, as applicable.					
13. Determined course of action for treatment.					
14. Explained planned treatment to client.					

Notes

14-2

Post-Service Procedure

A. Advise Clients and Promote Products

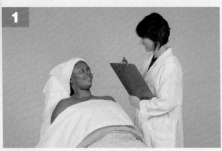

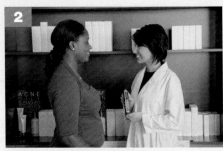

1 Before the client leaves your treatment area, ask her how she feels and if she enjoyed the service. Explain the conditions of her skin and your ideas about how to improve them. Be sure to ask if she has any questions or anything else she wishes to discuss. Be receptive and listen. Never be defensive. Determine a plan for future visits. Give the client ideas to think over for the next visit.

2 Advise client about proper home-care and explain how the recommended professional products will help to improve any skin conditions that are present. This is the time to discuss your retail product recommendations. Explain that these products are important and how to use them.

B. Schedule Next Appointment and Thank Client

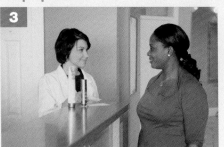

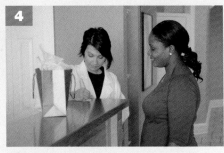

3 Escort the client to the reception desk and write up a service ticket for the client that includes the service provided, recommend home-care, and the next visit/service that needs to be scheduled. Place all recommended professional retail home-care products on counter for the client. Review the service ticket and the product recommendations with your client.

4 After the client has paid for her service and take-home products, ask if you can schedule her next appointment. Set up the date, time, and type of service for this next appointment, write the information on your business card, and give the card to the client.

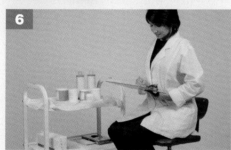

5 Thank the client for the opportunity to work with her. Express an interest in working with her in the future. Invite her to contact you should she have any questions or concerns about the service provided. If the client seems apprehensive, offer to call her in a day or two in order to check-in with her about any issues she may have. Genuinely wish her well, shake her hand, and wish her a great day.

6 Be sure to record service information, observations, and product recommendations on the client record, and be sure you return it to the proper place for filing.

At the End of the Day

1 Put on a fresh pair of gloves to protect yourself from contact with soiled linens and implements.

2 Turn off all equipment.

3 Remove all dirty laundry from the hamper. Spray the hamper with a disinfectant aerosol spray or wipe it down with disinfectant. Mildew grows easily in hampers.

4 Remove all dirty spatulas, used brushes, and other utensils. Most of these should have been removed between clients during the day.

5 Thoroughly clean and disinfect all multiuse tools and implements.

6 Wipe down all counters, the facial chair, machines, and other furniture with an approved disinfectant. The magnifying lamp should be cleaned on both sides in the same manner.

7 Replenish the room with fresh linens, spatulas, utensils, and other supplies so it is ready for the next day.

8 Change disinfection solution.

9 Maintain vaporizer as necessary.

10 Check the room for dirt, smudges, or dust on the walls, on the baseboards, in corners, or on air vents. Vacuum and mop the room with a disinfectant.

11 Replenish any empty jars. If you are reusing jars for dispensing creams from a bulk container, always use up the entire content of the small jar and thoroughly cleanse the jar before replenishing. Never add cream to a partially used jar. Rinse the empty jar well with hot water and then disinfect, rinsing thoroughly. Allow the jar to dry before refilling.

12 Empty waste containers. Replace with clean trash liners.

14-2

Rubrics are used in education for organizing and interpreting data gathered from observations of student performance. It is a clearly developed scoring document used to differentiate between levels of development in a specific skill performance or behavior. Rubrics are provided in this supplement for use as either a self-assessment tool to aid the student in behavior development or as an educator assessment tool to determine competence. Space is provided to record steps needed for further growth and improvement.

Performance is evaluated according to the following scale:

1 **Development Opportunity:** There is little or no evidence of competency; assistance is needed; performance includes multiple errors.

2 **Fundamental:** There is beginning evidence of competency; task is completed alone; performance includes few errors.

3 **Competent:** There is detailed and consistent evidence of competency; task is completed alone; performance includes rare errors.

4 **Strength:** There is detailed evidence of highly creative, inventive, mature presence of competency.

Space is provided for comments to assist you in improving your performance and achieving a higher rating.

Post-Service Procedure Assessment

PERFORMANCE ASSESSED	1	2	3	4	IMPROVEMENT PLAN
Advise Clients and Promote Products					
1. Before client left treatment area, asked how he/she felt about the service.					
2. Explained conditions of the skin and suggestions for improvement.					
3. Asked client if there were any questions.					
4. Was receptive and listened attentively.					
5. Determined a plan for future visits.					
6. Gave client ideas to consider for next visit.					
7. Advised client about proper home-care with emphasis on professional products.					
8. Discussed retail recommendations.					
9. Explained how to use home-care products.					
10. Escorted client to reception desk.					
11. Wrote up client ticket.					
12. Placed recommended retail home-care products on counter.					
13. Reviewed service ticket and product recommendations with client.					
14. Scheduled next appointment.					
15. Wrote the appointment information on business card and gave it to client.					
16. Thanked client for the opportunity to work with him/her.					

PERFORMANCE ASSESSED	1	2	3	4	IMPROVEMENT PLAN
17. Expressed an interest in working with client in future.					
18. Invited client to contact esthetician if he/she has questions or concerns.					
19. Offered to call client about any potential issues.					
20. Wished client well and shook hands.					
21. Recorded service information, observations, and product recommendations on client record.					
22. Properly filed the client record.					

End of the Day Cleanup

PERFORMANCE ASSESSED	1	2	3	4	IMPROVEMENT PLAN
1. Put on fresh gloves.					
2. Turned off all equipment.					
3. Removed dirty laundry from hamper.					
4. Sprayed hamper with a disinfectant aerosol spray and wiped it down with disinfectant.					
5. Removed all dirty spatulas, used brushes, and other utensils.					
6. Cleaned and disinfected all multiuse tools and equipment.					
7. Wiped down all counters, facial chair, machines, and furniture with an approved disinfectant.					
8. Cleaned magnifying lamp on both sides with disinfectant.					
9. Replenished room with fresh linens, spatulas, utensils, and other supplies.					
10. Changed disinfectant solution.					
11. Maintained vaporizer as necessary.					
12. Checked room for dirt, smudges, or dust on walls, baseboards, corners, and air vents.					
13. Vacuumed or swept and mopped room with a disinfectant.					
14. Sprayed air with a disinfectant aerosol spray.					
15. Rinsed empty jars with hot water.					
16. Disinfected empty jars.					
17. Allowed jars to dry before refilling.					
18. Replenished product in fresh, clean jars.					
19. Emptied waste containers.					
20. Replaced waste container with clean liner.					

14-2

14-3 & 14-4

IMPLEMENTS AND MATERIALS

- Roll of cotton
- Bowl
- Water
- Disinfectant
- Covered container or sealable plastic bag for storage

Preparation: Making Cleansing Pads and Butterfly Eye Pads

Preparation of Cotton Pads and Compresses

If prepackaged 4" × 4" (10 cm × 10 cm) esthetic wipes or sponges are not available, cotton pads can be made from a roll of cotton. You can prepare all cotton cleansing pads, eye pads, and the cotton compress pads that are used in a facial before the treatment begins. In a busy salon, the esthetician should check the appointment book at the beginning of each work day to see how many appointments are booked for that day. To save time, enough pads and compresses can then be made for the entire day if they are kept clean. Store pads and compresses in a covered container.

Remove enough pads from the container before each treatment and place them in a bowl that is kept within easy reach during the facial treatment. For each client, you may need a minimum of one pair of eye pads, one cotton compress mask, and four to six cleansing pads. The pads and compresses that are not used on the day they are made can be stored safely in an airtight, covered container or placed in a plastic bag and refrigerated for use the next day.

Notes

14-3

Making Cleansing Pads

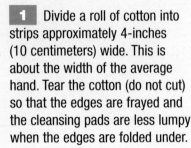
ON DVD

IMPLEMENTS
AND MATERIALS

- Roll of cotton
- Bowl
- Water
- Disinfectant
- Covered container or sealable plastic bag for storage

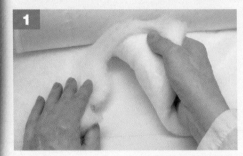

1 Divide a roll of cotton into strips approximately 4-inches (10 centimeters) wide. This is about the width of the average hand. Tear the cotton (do not cut) so that the edges are frayed and the cleansing pads are less lumpy when the edges are folded under.

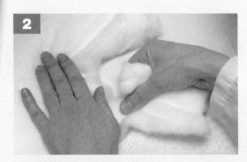

2 To make cleansing pads, hold one of the cotton strips in one hand and pull downward with the other hand until the cotton tears, making a cotton square approximately 4-inches (10 centimeters) wide by 5-inches (12.5 centimeters) long. Four to six of these pieces will be needed for each facial treatment.

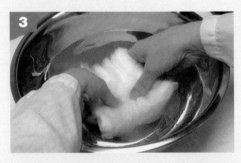

3 Submerge the cotton in water while supporting the pad with your fingers.

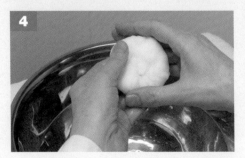

4 Tuck the edges of the cotton under while turning it in your hands. Place the round pad in the palm of your hand, placing the other palm over the pad. Squeeze out excess water from the pad.

Rubrics are used in education for organizing and interpreting data gathered from observations of student performance. It is a clearly developed scoring document used to differentiate between levels of development in a specific skill performance or behavior. Rubrics are provided in this supplement for use as either a self-assessment tool to aid the student in behavior development or as an educator assessment tool to determine competence. Space is provided to record steps needed for further growth and improvement.

Performance is evaluated according to the following scale:

1   **Development Opportunity:** There is little or no evidence of competency; assistance is needed; performance includes multiple errors.

2   **Fundamental:** There is beginning evidence of competency; task is completed alone; performance includes few errors.

3   **Competent:** There is detailed and consistent evidence of competency; task is completed alone; performance includes rare errors.

4   **Strength:** There is detailed evidence of highly creative, inventive, mature presence of competency.

Space is provided for comments to assist you in improving your performance and achieving a higher rating.

Making Cleansing Pads Assessment

PERFORMANCE ASSESSED	1	2	3	4	IMPROVEMENT PLAN
Procedure					
1. Divided roll of cotton into 4" (10cm) wide strips.					
2. Tore cotton so edges were frayed.					
3. Smoothed cotton to remove lumps.					
4. Tore cotton strip into sections approximately 4" (10cm) wide by 5" (12.5 cm) long.					
5. Submerged cotton pad in water while supporting pad with fingers.					
6. Tucked edges of cotton under while turning it in hands.					
7. Placed round pad in palm of hand.					
8. Placed other palm over pad.					
9. Squeezed out excess water from pad.					

14-3

IMPLEMENTS AND MATERIALS

- Roll of cotton
- Bowl
- Water
- Disinfectant
- Covered container or sealable plastic bag for storage

Making Butterfly Eye Pads

ON DVD ►

Eye pads can be made from either 4" × 4" (10 cm × 10 cm) cotton squares, prepackaged round cotton pads, or pieces of cotton. There are two types of eye pads: round and butterfly. Both styles of eye pads are correct, and the choice of which to use is up to the esthetician. The pads should be large enough to cover the entire eye area, but not so large that they interfere with product application or treatment. The advantage of the butterfly pad over the round pad is that it will not fall off of the eyes as easily. Round eye pads are made following the same procedure as for round cleansing pads, but the cotton piece should measure about 2½" × 2½" (6.25 cm × 6.25 cm).

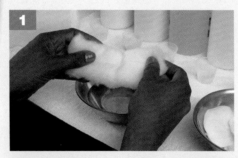

1 Dip a piece of cotton measuring approximately 2" × 6" (5 cm × 15 cm) into the water.

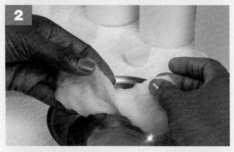

2 Twist the cotton in the center with a one-half turn.

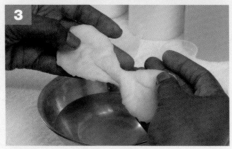

3 Fold the pad in half and squeeze out the excess water.

Optional: Take a prepackaged esthetics square 4" × 4" (10 cm × 10 cm) pad, unfold lengthwise, and twist it in the middle.

Clean-Up

- **Perform** **5-2** Aseptic Procedure PAGE 6

- **Complete** **14-2** Post-Service Procedure PAGE 22

© Milady, a part of Cengage Learning. Photography by Paul Castle, Castle Photography.

Rubrics are used in education for organizing and interpreting data gathered from observations of student performance. It is a clearly developed scoring document used to differentiate between levels of development in a specific skill performance or behavior. Rubrics are provided in this supplement for use as either a self-assessment tool to aid the student in behavior development or as an educator assessment tool to determine competence. Space is provided to record steps needed for further growth and improvement.

Performance is evaluated according to the following scale:

1 **Development Opportunity:** There is little or no evidence of competency; assistance is needed; performance includes multiple errors.

2 **Fundamental:** There is beginning evidence of competency; task is completed alone; performance includes few errors.

3 **Competent:** There is detailed and consistent evidence of competency; task is completed alone; performance includes rare errors.

4 **Strength:** There is detailed evidence of highly creative, inventive, mature presence of competency.

Space is provided for comments to assist you in improving your performance and achieving a higher rating

14-4

Making Butterfly Eye Pads Assessment

PERFORMANCE ASSESSED	1	2	3	4	IMPROVEMENT PLAN
Procedure					
1. Tore a 6" (15 cm) wide strip from the roll of cotton.					
2. Tore strip into 2" (5 cm) sections.					
3. Tore cotton so edges were frayed.					
4. Smoothed cotton to remove lumps.					
5. Submerged cotton strip in water while supporting pad with fingers.					
6. Twisted cotton strip in center with a one-half turn.					
7. Folded strip in half.					
8. Squeezed out excess water from pad.					

15-1

Eye Makeup and Lipstick Removal

ON DVD ▶

IMPLEMENTS AND MATERIALS

- Disinfectant
- Hand sanitizer/antibacterial soap
- Covered waste container
- Bowl
- Spatula
- Hand towels
- Headband
- Clean linens
- Bolster

Single-use Items

- Gloves
- Cotton pads
- Cotton rounds
- Cotton swabs
- Plastic bag
- Paper towels
- Tissues

Products

- Eye makeup remover or cleanser
- Facial cleanser

Preparation

- **Perform** **14-1** PROCEDURE **Pre-Service Procedure** PAGE 16

Procedure

Eye Makeup Removal

Note: If the client is wearing contacts, do not remove the eye makeup. Be especially gentle when cleansing the eyes because the skin around the eyes is very sensitive and can become irritated. Do not get cleanser into the eyes.

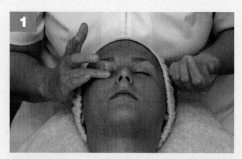

1 Apply a small amount of cleanser.

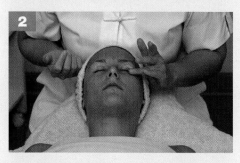

2 With the middle and ring fingers, apply the cleanser to the eyelids with gentle downward strokes. Use downward movements with the cleansing pad to cleanse the eyelid and lashes. Gently rinse with cotton pads.

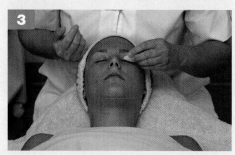

3 Repeat this step as necessary to remove eye makeup. While cleansing the eyes, rotate the pad to provide a clean, unused surface.

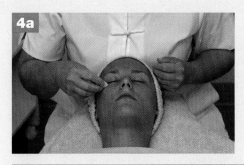

4a Rinse under the eyes sweeping in towards the nose. Remove any makeup underneath the eyes and along the lash line with a cotton swab or pad. Place the edge of the pad under the lower lashes at the outside corner of the eyes, and slide the pad toward the inner corner of the eyes. The mascara will gradually work loose and can be wiped clean. Always be gentle around the eyes; never rub or stretch the skin, as it is very delicate and thin.

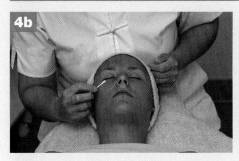

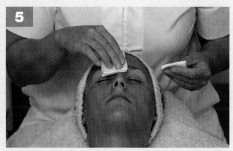

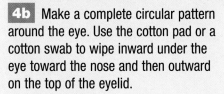

4b Make a complete circular pattern around the eye. Use the cotton pad or a cotton swab to wipe inward under the eye toward the nose and then outward on the top of the eyelid.

5 Rinse the eye area with plain water to remove the eye makeup remover. Make sure the remover is rinsed off thoroughly.

Lipstick Removal

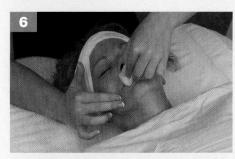

6 To remove lipstick, apply eye makeup remover or a cleanser to a damp cotton pad or tissue and remove the client's lipstick. Use a small amount and do not get cleanser in the mouth—it does not taste good.

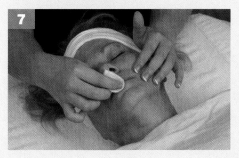

7 With the index and middle finger (either the left or right side) of one hand, hold on next to the outside edge of the lips to keep the skin taut so it does not move around; then remove the cleanser with the other hand using even strokes from the corners of the lips toward the center from both sides.

8 Repeat the procedure on the other side until the lips are clean.

Post-Service

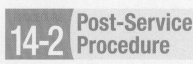

• **Complete** **14-2** **Post-Service Procedure** PAGE 22

15-1

Rubrics are used in education for organizing and interpreting data gathered from observations of student performance. It is a clearly developed scoring document used to differentiate between levels of development in a specific skill performance or behavior. Rubrics are provided in this supplement for use as either a self-assessment tool to aid the student in behavior development or as an educator assessment tool to determine competence. Space is provided to record steps needed for further growth and improvement.

Performance is evaluated according to the following scale:

1 Development Opportunity: There is little or no evidence of competency; assistance is needed; performance includes multiple errors.

2 Fundamental: There is beginning evidence of competency; task is completed alone; performance includes few errors.

3 Competent: There is detailed and consistent evidence of competency; task is completed alone; performance includes rare errors.

4 Strength: There is detailed evidence of highly creative, inventive, mature presence of competency.

Space is provided for comments to assist you in improving your performance and achieving a higher rating.

Eye Makeup and Lipstick Removal Assessment

PERFORMANCE ASSESSED	1	2	3	4	IMPROVEMENT PLAN
Preparation					
Performed standard pre-service procedure.					
Eye Makeup Removal Procedure					
1. Applied a small amount of cleanser.					
2. Used middle and ring fingers of right hand, applied cleanser to eyelid with downward strokes.					
3. Cleansed eyelid and lashes with cleansing pad applied in downward movements.					
4. Gently rinsed with cotton pads.					
5. Repeated cleansing steps as necessary.					
6. Rotated pad while cleansing to provide a clean, unused surface.					
7. Rinsed under the eyes sweeping inward toward the nose.					
8. Placed the edge of the pad under lower lashes at the outside corner of the eyes.					
9. Slid the pad toward the inner corner of the eyes.					
10. Removed any makeup under the eyes.					
11. Did not rub or stretch the skin.					
12. Using cotton pad or swab, completed the circular pattern.					
13. Rinsed the eye area with plain water to remove product thoroughly.					

PERFORMANCE ASSESSED	1	2	3	4	IMPROVEMENT PLAN
Lipstick Removal Procedure					
1. Applied small amount of cleanser to damp cotton pad or tissue.					
2. With index and middle finger of one hand, held outside edge of the lips taut.					
3. Removed lipstick with even strokes from corners of lips toward center.					
4. Repeated procedure on the opposite side of lips.					
5. Continued until lips were clean.					

Notes

_____

_____

_____

_____

_____

_____

_____

_____

_____

_____

_____

_____

_____

_____

_____

_____

_____

_____

15-1

Applying a Cleansing Product

IMPLEMENTS AND MATERIALS

- Disinfectant
- Hand sanitizer/antibacterial soap
- Covered waste container
- Bowl
- Spatula
- Facial towels
- Headband
- Clean linens
- Bolster

Single-use Items

- Gloves
- Cotton pads
- Cotton rounds
- Cotton swabs
- Plastic bag
- Paper towels
- Tissues

Products

- Eye makeup remover or cleanser
- Facial cleanser
- Toner
- Moisturizer

The following method of application is used when applying cleansers, massage creams, treatment creams, and protective products. Most product removal requires rinsing each area at least three times. If possible, use both hands at the same time for a more even and efficient technique. Use either circular motions or straight, even strokes for cleansing.

Preparation

- **Perform** 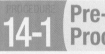 **14-1** **Pre-Service Procedure** PAGE 16

Procedure

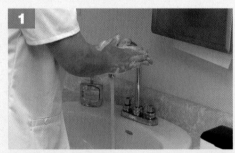

1 Cleanse the hands and apply gloves before touching the client's face. Apply warm towels. After checking the temperature, apply one towel to the décolleté and one to the face. Leave on at least 1 minute and then remove.

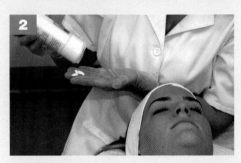

2 Apply approximately one-half teaspoon of the product to the fingers or palms of the hand. Water-soluble cleansing lotion is preferred over foamy cleansers when cleansing the face because it can be removed easier with moistened cotton pads or sponges.

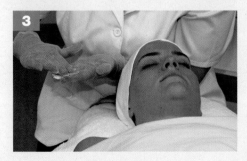

3 Use circular motions to distribute the product onto the fingertips. You are now ready to apply the product to the client's décolleté, neck, and face. Cleanse each area using six passes. If starting on the décolleté, start in the center and work out to the sides moving up to the neck. Be guided by your instructor.

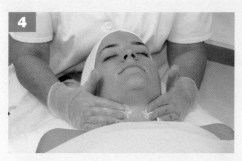

4 Start applying a small amount of the product by placing both hands, palms down, on the neck. Slide hands back toward the ears until the pads of the fingers rest at a point directly beneath the earlobes. While applying the product, it is suggested that hands are not lifted from the client's face until you are finished.

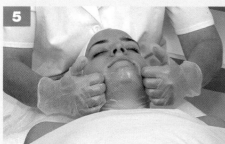

5 Reverse the hand, with the back of the fingers now resting on the skin, and slide the fingers along the jawline to the chin.

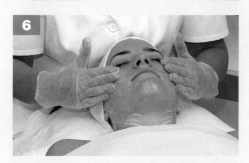

6 Reverse the hands again and slide the fingers back over the cheeks and center of the face until the pads of the fingers come to rest directly in front of the ears.

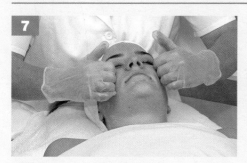

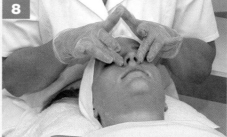

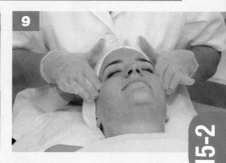

7 Reverse the hands again, and slide the fingers forward over the cheekbones to the nose. Cleanse the upper lip area under the nose with sideways strokes from the center area moving outward. Then slide up to the sides of the nose.

8 With the pads of the middle fingers, make small, circular motions on the top of the nose and on each side of the nose. Avoid pushing the product into the nose.

9 Slide the fingers up to the forehead and outward toward the temples, pausing with a slight pressure on the temples. Slide fingers across the forehead using circles or long strokes from side to side.

10 Continue to remove the product in Procedure 15–3, Removing Products.

15-2

Rubrics are used in education for organizing and interpreting data gathered from observations of student performance. It is a clearly developed scoring document used to differentiate between levels of development in a specific skill performance or behavior. Rubrics are provided in this supplement for use as either a self-assessment tool to aid the student in behavior development or as an educator assessment tool to determine competence. Space is provided to record steps needed for further growth and improvement.

Performance is evaluated according to the following scale:

1   **Development Opportunity:** There is little or no evidence of competency; assistance is needed; performance includes multiple errors.

2   **Fundamental:** There is beginning evidence of competency; task is completed alone; performance includes few errors.

3   **Competent:** There is detailed and consistent evidence of competency; task is completed alone; performance includes rare errors.

4   **Strength:** There is detailed evidence of highly creative, inventive, mature presence of competency.

Space is provided for comments to assist you in improving your performance and achieving a higher rating.

Applying a Cleansing Product Assessment

PERFORMANCE ASSESSED	1	2	3	4	IMPROVEMENT PLAN
Preparation					
Performed standard pre-service procedure.					
Procedure					
1. Cleansed own hands.					
2. Applied gloves.					
3. Applied warm towel to décolleté.					
4. Applied warm towel to face.					
5. Applied cleanser to fingertips.					
6. Used circular motion to distribute product on fingertips.					
7. Applied product to client's décolleté, neck, and face.					
8. Placed both hands, palms down, on neck.					
9. Slid hands back toward ears until pads of fingers rested beneath earlobes.					
10. Slid backs of fingers along jawline to chin.					
11. Slid pads of fingers back over cheeks to rest directly in front of ears.					
12. Slid backs of fingers forward over cheekbones to the nose.					
13. Cleansed upper lip area under nose with sideways strokes.					
14. Slid up to sides of the nose.					
15 Using pads of middle fingers, made small circular movements on top and sides of nose.					

PERFORMANCE ASSESSED	1	2	3	4	IMPROVEMENT PLAN
16. Slid fingers to the forehead and outward to temples, paused with slight pressure on temples.					
17. Slid fingers across forehead using circles or long strokes from side to side.					

Notes

_____

_____

_____

_____

_____

_____

_____

_____

_____

_____

_____

_____

_____

_____

_____

_____

_____

_____

15-2

15-3

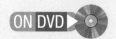

Removing Products

IMPLEMENTS AND MATERIALS

- Disinfectant
- Hand sanitizer/antibacterial soap
- Covered waste container
- Bowl
- Spatula
- Facial towels
- Headband
- Clean linens
- Bolster

Single-use Items

- Gloves
- Cotton pads
- Cotton rounds
- Cotton swabs
- Plastic bag
- Paper towels
- Tissues

Products

- Eye makeup remover or cleanser
- Facial cleanser
- Toner
- Moisturizer

To remove products, rinse each area at least three to six times. Some estheticians prefer to use wet cotton pads or disposable facial sponges when removing product. Others prefer to use towels. Both methods are correct and equally professional, and many estheticians use both methods. For example, an esthetician who usually uses the sponges will use cotton pads when working on acne skin. Even when using sponges, an esthetician may need cotton pads during the treatment for eye pads or removing blackheads.

Facial movements are generally done in an upward and outward direction from the center to the edges of the face. Under the eyes, it is usually inward to avoid tugging on the eye area.

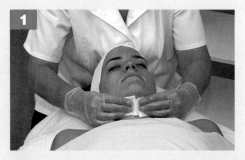

1 Starting at the décolleté, cleanse sideways and up to the neck. Cleanse the neck using upward strokes. To keep the pad from slipping from the hand, pinch the edge of the pad between the thumb and upper part of the forefinger. It is important that most of the surface of the pad remain in contact with the skin. Do not exert pressure on the Adam's apple in the center of the neck.

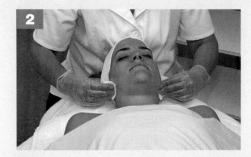

2 Place the pad directly under the chin and slide the pad along the jawline, stopping directly under the ear. Repeat the movement on the other side of the face. Alternate back and forth three times on each side of the face, or do the movement concurrently by using both hands at the same time.

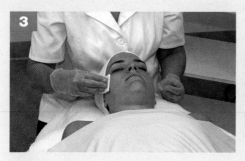

3 Starting at the jawline, use upward movements to cleanse the cheeks.

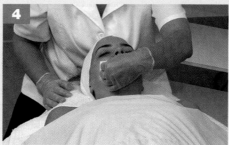

4 Continuing the upward movement and cross over the chin to the other cheek if you are only using one hand.

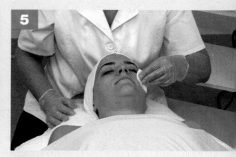

5 Continue the cleansing movement with approximately six strokes on each cheek.

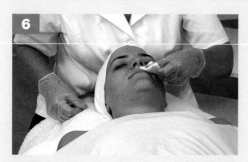

6 Cleanse the area directly underneath the nose by using downward and sideways strokes. Start at the center and work outward toward the corners of the mouth. Rinse at least three times on each side of the face.

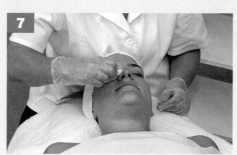

7 Starting on the bridge of the nose, cleanse the sides of the nose and the area directly next to it. Use light, outward movements.

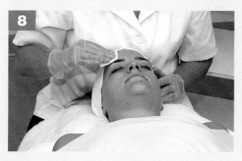

8 Place the pads flat on the center of the forehead, and slide them outward to the temples. Apply a slight pressure on the pressure points of the temples. Repeat the movement three times on each side of the forehead.

9 Check the face to make sure there is no residue left on the skin. Feather over the areas of the face with the finger tips to check that it is well rinsed.

Post-Service

- **Complete** 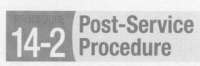 **PROCEDURE 14-2 Post-Service Procedure** PAGE 22

15-3

Rubrics are used in education for organizing and interpreting data gathered from observations of student performance. It is a clearly developed scoring document used to differentiate between levels of development in a specific skill performance or behavior. Rubrics are provided in this supplement for use as either a self-assessment tool to aid the student in behavior development or as an educator assessment tool to determine competence. Space is provided to record steps needed for further growth and improvement.

Performance is evaluated according to the following scale:

1   **Development Opportunity:** There is little or no evidence of competency; assistance is needed; performance includes multiple errors.

2   **Fundamental:** There is beginning evidence of competency; task is completed alone; performance includes few errors.

3   **Competent:** There is detailed and consistent evidence of competency; task is completed alone; performance includes rare errors.

4   **Strength:** There is detailed evidence of highly creative, inventive, mature presence of competency.

Space is provided for comments to assist you in improving your performance and achieving a higher rating.

Removing Products Assessment

PERFORMANCE ASSESSED	1	2	3	4	IMPROVEMENT PLAN
Preparation					
Performed standard pre-service procedure.					
Procedure					
1. Starting at décolleté, cleansed sideways and up to the neck.					
2. Cleansed neck using upward strokes.					
3. To prevent slipping, pinched edge of pad between thumb and forefinger.					
4. Did not exert pressure on Adam's apple.					
5. Placed pad directly under chin and slid along jawline, stopping under ear.					
6. Repeated movement on opposite side of face.					
7. Alternated back and forth three times on each side of face OR performed movement concurrently with both hands.					
8. Started at jawline and cleansed cheeks using upward movements.					
9. Continued upward movement, crossed over chin to other cheek.					
10. Continued cleansing with approximately six strokes on each cheek.					
11. Cleansed area beneath nose using downward and sideways strokes.					
12. Started at center and worked outward towards corner of mouth.					
13. Rinsed at least three times on each side of face.					

PERFORMANCE ASSESSED	1	2	3	4	IMPROVEMENT PLAN
14. Started at bridge of nose and cleansed sides of nose and area directly next to it.					
15. Placed pads flat on center of forehead and slid outward to temple.					
16. Applied slight pressure at temples.					
17. Repeated movement three times on each side of forehead.					
18. Ensured there was no remaining residue on the skin.					

Notes

_____

_____

_____

_____

_____

_____

_____

_____

_____

_____

_____

_____

_____

_____

_____

_____

_____

IMPLEMENTS AND MATERIALS

Equipment
- Facial equipment (towel warmer, steamer, mag light)

Supplies
- Disinfectant
- Hand sanitizer/antibacterial soap
- Covered waste container
- Bowls
- Spatulas
- Fan and mask brush
- Implements
- Distilled water
- Sharps container
- Hand towels
- Clean linens
- Blanket
- Headband
- Client wrap
- Bolster
- Client charts

Single-use Items
- Cotton pads
- Cotton rounds
- Cotton swabs
- Paper towels
- Tissue
- Gloves/finger cots
- Sealable plastic bag

Products
- Cleanser
- Exfoliant
- Masks
- Massage lotion
- Toner
- Moisturizer
- Sunscreen
- Optional: serums, eye cream, lip balm, extraction supplies

The Basic Step-by-Step Facial

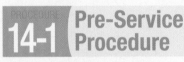

ON DVD

Now that you have practiced the preliminary steps and cleansing, it is time to put it all together in a complete facial. The steps for performing a basic facial treatment are listed here. Facial procedures vary, so be guided by your instructor.

While not shown, wearing gloves may be required while performing facial services in your region.

Preparation

- **Perform** **14-1** **Pre-Service Procedure** PAGE 16

Procedure

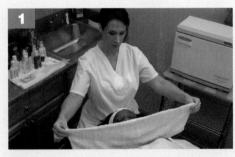

1 **Cleanse your hands and apply warm towels.** After checking the temperature, apply one towel to the décolleté and one to the face.

To apply warm towels: Hold the ends of the towels with both hands on either side of the face. Lay the center of the towel on the chin and drape each side across the face with the towel edges draped over to the opposite corner across the forehead. To remove, lift each end and remove. For product removal: use the towels over the hands as mitts. Be guided by your instructor on this method.

Optional: Remove eye makeup and lipstick. If your client has no makeup, skip this part and proceed to step 2. Remember to ask about contact lenses before putting product on the eyes. If the client is wearing contacts, do not remove the eye makeup.

2 Cleanse

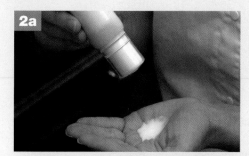

2a Remove about one-half teaspoon of cleanser from the container (with a clean spatula if it is not a squirt-top or pump-type lid). Place it on the fingertips or in the palm and then apply a small amount to your fingertips. This conserves the amount of product you use.

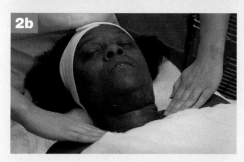

2b Starting at the neck or décolleté and with a sweeping movement, use both hands to spread the cleanser upward and outward on the chin, jaws, cheeks, and temples. Spread the cleanser down the nose and along its sides and bridge. Continue to the upper lip area. Cleanse the upper lip area under the nose with sideways strokes from the center area moving outward.

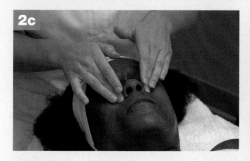

2c Make small, circular movements with the fingertips around the nostrils and sides of the nose. Continue with upward-sweeping movements between the brows and across the forehead to the temples.

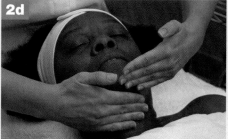

2d Apply more cleanser to the neck and chest with long, outward strokes. Cleanse the area in small, circular motions from the center of the chest and neck toward the outside, moving upward. Try to use both hands at the same time on each side when applying or removing product.

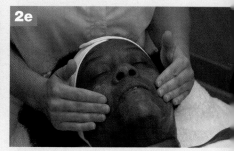

2e Visually divide the face into left and right halves from the center. Continue moving upward with circular motions on the face from the chin and cheeks, and up toward the forehead using both hands, one on each side.

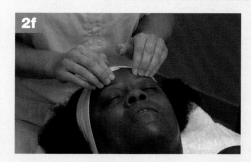

2f Starting at the center of the forehead, continue with the circular pattern out to the temples. Move the fingertips lightly in a circle around the eyes to the temples and then back to the center of the forehead. Lift your hands slowly off of the face when you finish cleansing.

15-4

15-4 The Basic Step-by-Step Facial (continued)

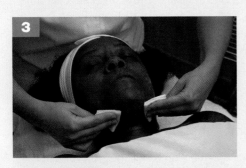

3 **Remove the cleanser.** Using moist cotton pads or disposable facial sponges, start at the neck or forehead and follow the contours of the face. Move up or down the face in a consistent pattern, depending on where you start according to the instructor's procedures. Remove all the cleanser from one area of the face before proceeding to the next. (Under the nostrils, use downward strokes when applying or removing products to avoid pushing product up the nose. This is uncomfortable and will make the client tense.) Blot your hands on a clean towel, and touch the face with dry fingertips to make sure there is no residue left.

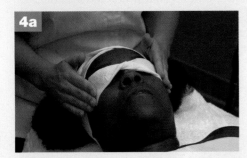

4a **Analyze the skin.**

Cover the client's eyes with eye pads.

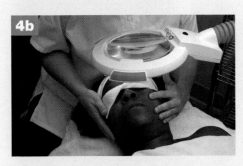

4b Position the magnifying light where you want it before starting the facial, so that you can swing it over easily to line up over the face. Note the skin type and condition, and feel the texture of the skin.

Optional: Cleanse the face again. Some treatment protocols do not include this second cleansing. Be guided by your instructor.

Optional: If exfoliation is part of the service, it could be done at this time before steaming. If eyebrow arching is needed, it could be done either at this time or following the steam and extractions to avoid irritation from the steam. Be careful what you apply to freshly waxed areas.

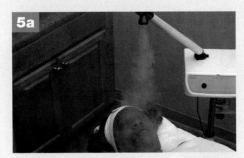

5a **Steam the face.**

Preheat the steamer before you need it. Check that the water level is at the appropriate fill line. Turn it on, wait for it to start steaming, and then turn on the second ozone button if applicable while steaming.

Caution: Keep the steam facing away from the client until it is steaming to avoid potential spitting of water which may happen if the machine is overfilled or not maintained properly.

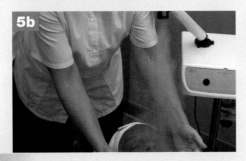

5b Check to make sure the steamer is not too close to the client (approximately 18 inches [45 centimeters] away) and that it is steaming the face evenly. If you hold your hands close to the sides of the client's face, you can feel if the steam is reaching both sides of the face. Steam for approximately 5 to 10 minutes.

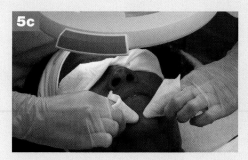

5c Turn off the steamer immediately after use. If using towels in place of steam, remember to test them for the correct temperature. Ask the client if she is comfortable with the temperature. Towels are left on for approximately 2 minutes. Steam or warm towels should be used carefully on couperose skin.

Optional: Extractions are done immediately after the steam, while the skin is still warm. Refer to the extractions section of this chapter to incorporate this step into your basic facial procedure if it is applicable to your facility.

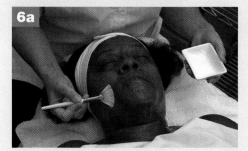

6a Massage the face.

Select a water-soluble massage cream or product appropriate to the client's skin type. Use the same procedure as you did for product application to apply the massage cream to the face, neck, shoulders, and chest. Apply the warmed product in long, slow strokes with fingers or a soft fan brush, moving in a set pattern.

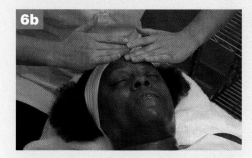

6b Perform the massage as directed.

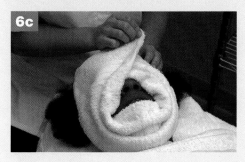

6c Remove the massage cream. Use warm towels or cleansing pads and follow the same procedure as for removing other products or cleanser.

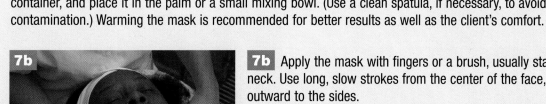

7a Choose a mask formulated for the client's skin condition. Remove the mask from its container, and place it in the palm or a small mixing bowl. (Use a clean spatula, if necessary, to avoid contamination.) Warming the mask is recommended for better results as well as the client's comfort.

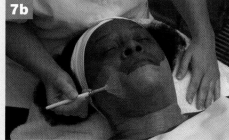

7b Apply the mask with fingers or a brush, usually starting at the neck. Use long, slow strokes from the center of the face, moving outward to the sides.

15-4

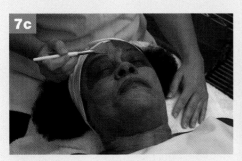

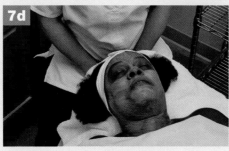

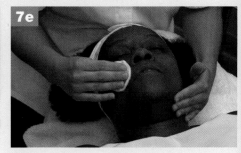

7c Proceed to the jawline and apply the mask on the face from the center outward. Avoid the eye area unless the mask is appropriate for that area.

7d Allow the mask to remain on the face for approximately 7 to 10 minutes.

7e Remove the mask with towels, followed by wet cotton pads or sponges.

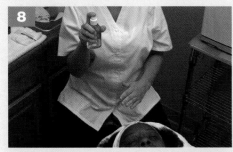

8 Apply the toner product appropriate for the skin type.

Note: Serums as well as eye and lip creams are optional for application before the final moisturizer.

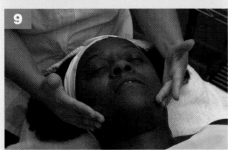

9 Apply a moisturizer (and an additional sunscreen as appropriate).

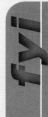

fyi Never remove products from containers with your fingers. Always use a spatula. Do not touch fingertips to lids or openings of containers. Clean and disinfect product containers after each service.

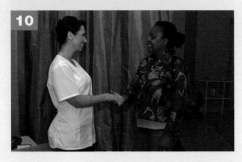

10 End the facial by washing your hands and quietly letting the client know you are finished. Give the client instructions for getting dressed. Have the client come out to the reception area when they are ready to discuss the home-care products and regime.

Post-Service

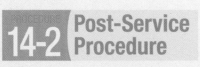

- **Complete** **14-2** Post-Service Procedure PAGE 22

FOCUS ON

Clients

The importance of following proper hygiene, health, and safety guidelines when giving facials cannot be overemphasized. As much as possible, wash your hands in the presence of your clients. When they see you doing this, they will have more confidence in your infection prevention.

Rubrics are used in education for organizing and interpreting data gathered from observations of student performance. It is a clearly developed scoring document used to differentiate between levels of development in a specific skill performance or behavior. Rubrics are provided in this supplement for use as either a self-assessment tool to aid the student in behavior development or as an educator assessment tool to determine competence. Space is provided to record steps needed for further growth and improvement.

Performance is evaluated according to the following scale:

1 Development Opportunity: There is little or no evidence of competency; assistance is needed; performance includes multiple errors.

2 Fundamental: There is beginning evidence of competency; task is completed alone; performance includes few errors.

3 Competent: There is detailed and consistent evidence of competency; task is completed alone; performance includes rare errors.

4 Strength: There is detailed evidence of highly creative, inventive, mature presence of competency.

Space is provided for comments to assist you in improving your performance and achieving a higher rating.

The Basic Step-by-Step Facial Assessment

PERFORMANCE ASSESSED	1	2	3	4	IMPROVEMENT PLAN
Preparation					
Completed standard pre-service procedure.					
Cleansing Procedure					
1. Cleansed own hands.					
2. Applied warm towel to décolleté.					
3. Applied warm towel to face.					
4. Removed eye makeup and lipstick, if applicable.					
5. Properly removed product with spatula (fingertips were never used).					
6. Applied cleanser to fingertips.					
7. Started at neck or décolleté and spread cleanser upward and outward on chin, jaws, cheeks, and temples.					
8. Spread cleanser down nose and along its sides and bridge.					
9. Cleansed upper lip area under nose with sideways strokes from center moving outward.					
10. Made small circular movements around nostrils and sides of nose.					
11. Continued upward-sweeping movements between brows and across forehead to temples.					
12. Cleansed neck and chest with circular motions from center toward outside, moving upward.					

15-4

PERFORMANCE ASSESSED	1	2	3	4	IMPROVEMENT PLAN
13. Continued moving upward with circular motions from the chin and cheeks toward forehead with both hands, one on each side.					
14. Started at center of forehead and continued with circular pattern to temples.					
15. Moved fingertips lightly in a circle around the eyes to the temples and back to center of forehead.					
16. Lifted hands slowly off face when cleansing was complete.					
17. Removed cleanser starting at neck or forehead and followed facial contours.					
18. Removed cleanser from one area of face before proceeding to the next.					
19. Ensured there was no remaining residue on skin.					
Skin Analysis					
1. Covered client's eyes with eye pads.					
2. Properly positioned magnifying light.					
3. Noted skin type, condition, and texture.					
Machine Steaming					
1. Preheated the steamer after checking water level.					
2. Turned on ozone button if applicable.					
3. Positioned steamer 18"(45 cm) away from face.					
4. Steamed face for 5 to 10 minutes.					
5. Turned off steamer after use.					
Towel Steaming					
1. Checked and confirmed towel temperature.					
2. Applied steaming towels to face.					
3. Steamed with towels for 2 minutes.					
4. Extractions were performed following steaming, if applicable.					
Massage					
1. Selected appropriate massage cream.					
2. Applied massage cream to face, neck, shoulders, and chest.					
3. Performed correct massage procedure.					
4. Removed massage cream using warm towels or cleansing pads.					

PERFORMANCE ASSESSED	1	2	3	4	IMPROVEMENT PLAN
Mask					
1. Chose appropriate mask formula.					
2. Properly warmed and removed mask.					
3. Applied mask with fingers or brush starting at neck using slow strokes from center of face, moving outward to sides.					
4. Continued applying mask from jawline outward.					
5. Eye area was avoided.					
6. Allowed mask to remain for 7 to 10 minutes.					
7. Removed mask with wet cotton pads, sponges, or towels.					
Tone and Moisturize					
1. Applied appropriate toner.					
2. Applied appropriate moisturizer.					
Completion					
1. Washed own hands.					
2. Informed client service was complete and gave instructions for dressing.					
3. Discussed home-care products and regimen.					
Post-Service					
Completed standard post-service, cleanup, and disinfection procedures.					

Notes

15-4

15-5

IMPLEMENTS AND MATERIALS

- Cotton roll
- Scissors
- Basin of warm water
- Product

Applying the Cotton Compress

ON DVD ▶ 💿

Note: This procedure is outdated but some licensing boards may still test on it.

Preparation

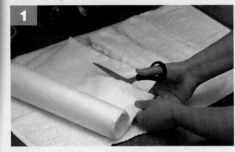

1 Prepare the cotton on a clean and disinfected work area.

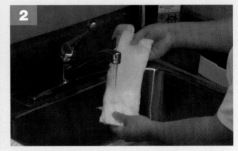

2 Wet and unfold the cotton strip, and carefully divide it lengthwise into three separate strips. Try to keep the thickness of each strip as even as possible.

Procedure

The steps for applying a cotton compress alone or over a mask are as follows:

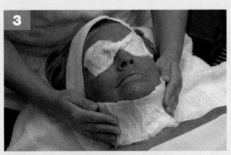

3 Secure eye pads on the client's eyes. Take the strip that feels the thinnest and mold it to the client's neck. Be sure the strip does not overlap on the underside of the chin and jawline.

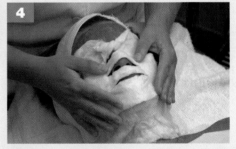

4 Place the center of the second strip of cotton (saving the thickest piece for last) on the chin, under the lower lip. Mold the cotton under the jaw, chin, and lower part of the cheeks. Leave breathing access by molding the strips around the tip of the nose.

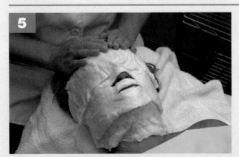

5 Place the third and thickest cotton strip over the upper portion of the face (eye pads remain in place). Carefully stretch the cotton.

Rubrics are used in education for organizing and interpreting data gathered from observations of student performance. It is a clearly developed scoring document used to differentiate between levels of development in a specific skill performance or behavior. Rubrics are provided in this supplement for use as either a self-assessment tool to aid the student in behavior development or as an educator assessment tool to determine competence. Space is provided to record steps needed for further growth and improvement.

Performance is evaluated according to the following scale:

1 **Development Opportunity:** There is little or no evidence of competency; assistance is needed; performance includes multiple errors.

2 **Fundamental:** There is beginning evidence of competency; task is completed alone; performance includes few errors.

3 **Competent:** There is detailed and consistent evidence of competency; task is completed alone; performance includes rare errors.

4 **Strength:** There is detailed evidence of highly creative, inventive, mature presence of competency.

Space is provided for comments to assist you in improving your performance and achieving a higher rating.

Applying the Cotton Compress Assessment

PERFORMANCE ASSESSED	1	2	3	4	IMPROVEMENT PLAN
Preparation					
1. Prepared the cotton.					
2. Wet cotton strip.					
3. Unfolded cotton strip.					
4. Divided cotton strip into three separate strips.					
5. Maintained uniform thickness for strips.					
Procedure					
1. Secured eye pads on client's eyes.					
2. Molded cotton strip to client's neck.					
3. Did not overlap neck strip on the underside of chin and jawline.					
4. Placed center of second cotton strip on chin under lower lip.					
5. Molded cotton under jaw, chin, and lower part of cheeks.					
6. Molded strips around tip of nose leaving breathing access.					
7. Placed a cotton strip over the upper portion of the face.					
8. Used care in stretching cotton.					

15-6

Removing the Cotton Compress

ON DVD ▶ ⊙

IMPLEMENTS
AND MATERIALS
- Cotton roll
- Cotton pads
- Ice cubes or face globes
- Waste container

1 **Optional step:** Massage over the surface of the compress mask with an ice cube or cool face globes if applicable, using circular movements. The ice will feel refreshing and will firm the skin. As the ice melts, the water seeps into the compress, helping to soften the mask underneath.

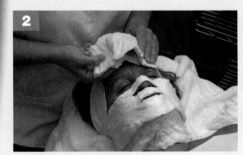

2 Starting on the upper part of the face, place the hands, palms down, on each side of the face. With one hand, slide the compress slowly toward the side of the face, picking up as much of the treatment mask as possible. The eye pads will come off at the same time and should be discarded.

3 Fold the strip in half, so that the side of the compress that has the treatment mask on it is inside and the compress strip has two clean surfaces. Squeeze the cotton over a waste container to remove any excess water.

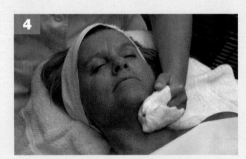

4 Tear a separate strip of wet cotton in half, wrapping around the first three fingers of the hand to form a cotton mitt. Use the cotton mitts to further remove remaining traces of the mask. If necessary, cotton pads, rather than finger mitts, can be used to cleanse the face.

Rubrics are used in education for organizing and interpreting data gathered from observations of student performance. It is a clearly developed scoring document used to differentiate between levels of development in a specific skill performance or behavior. Rubrics are provided in this supplement for use as either a self-assessment tool to aid the student in behavior development or as an educator assessment tool to determine competence. Space is provided to record steps needed for further growth and improvement.

Performance is evaluated according to the following scale:

1 **Development Opportunity:** There is little or no evidence of competency; assistance is needed; performance includes multiple errors.

2 **Fundamental:** There is beginning evidence of competency; task is completed alone; performance includes few errors.

3 **Competent:** There is detailed and consistent evidence of competency; task is completed alone; performance includes rare errors.

4 **Strength:** There is detailed evidence of highly creative, inventive, mature presence of competency.

Space is provided for comments to assist you in improving your performance and achieving a higher rating.

Removing the Cotton Compress Assessment

PERFORMANCE ASSESSED	1	2	3	4	IMPROVEMENT PLAN
Optional Step					
Massaged over surface of compress mask with ice cubes or cool face globes using circular movements.					
Procedure					
1. At upper part of face, placed hands, palms down, on each side of face.					
2. Using one hand, slid the compress slowly toward side of face.					
3. Picked up as much of treatment mask as possible.					
4. Removed eye pads simultaneously.					
5. Discarded eye pads.					
6. Folded compress in half with treatment mask on the inside.					
7. Discarded compresses.					
8. Tore a separate strip of wet cotton in half.					
9. Wrapped wet strip around first three fingers to form cotton mitt.					
10. Removed remaining traces of mask.					

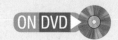
ON DVD

PROCEDURE
15-7

IMPLEMENTS AND MATERIALS

- Basin of water
- Cotton pads
- Gloves
- Astringent
- Sealable plastic bag
- Other appropriate facial supplies, products, and equipment

Extractions

Preparation

Preparing the Fingers for Comedone Extractions

If you are using 4" × 4" (10 cm × 10 cm) or 2" × 2" (5 cm × 5 cm) premade pads, apply astringent to pads (without oversaturating them) and wrap around fingers. If you are not using four premade pads, prepare cotton as follows. Always wear gloves during extractions.

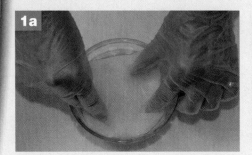
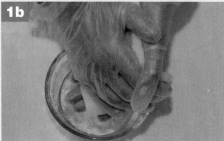

1 Dip strips of clean cotton in water and squeeze out the excess.

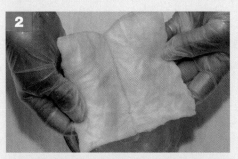

2 Unfold the pad and divide it into two thinner pieces. Place one-half of the pad back in the bowl that holds the cleansing pads. With astringent, lightly saturate the half of the pad you are holding. Squeeze out the excess astringent.

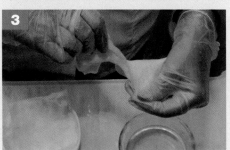

3 Tear small strips from the astringent-saturated cotton.

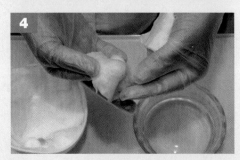

4 Wrap fingers with dampened pads. Wrap the strips smoothly around the end of each index finger. Repeat this step until the fingertips are well padded (approximately ⅛-inch [3 millimeters] thick).

Procedure

Performing Extractions

Prepare the client's skin. Extractions are performed during a treatment after the skin is warmed and prepared/softened with product. Never extract on unprepared dry, cold skin. Extraction procedures for different facial areas follow:

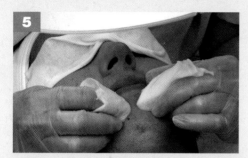

5 **Chin.** On a flat area, press down, under, in, and up. Work around the plug, pressing down, in, and up. Bring fingers in toward each other around the follicle without pinching.

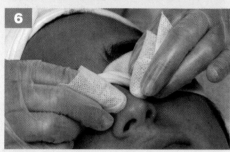

6 **Nose.** Slide fingers down each side of the nose, holding the nostril tissue firmly, but do not press down too firmly on the nose. The fingers on top do the sliding, while the other one holds close to the bottom of the follicle. Do not cut off the air flow to the nostrils.

7 **Cheeks.** Slide fingers together down the cheek, holding each section of the skin as you go. The lower hand holds and the other hand slides toward the lower hand.

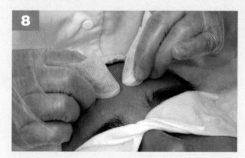

8 **Forehead; upper cheekbones.** Extract as on the chin: press down, in, and up.

Post-Service

• **Complete** **14-2** **Post-Service Procedure** PAGE 22

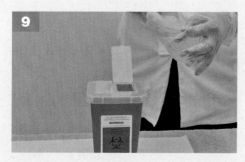

9 **Note:** Dispose of gloves and supplies properly. Change gloves to continue the facial treatment.

fyi

Extractions with Lancets

When a lesion is sealed over, as in old blackheads and closed comedones, a small-gauge needle or lancet is used for extraction. The lancet should be inserted at a 35-degree angle or parallel to the surface of the skin. Slowly insert the needle just under the top of the plug, lift the top off, and open it gently. Never put the needle down into the follicle because it is painful and could damage it. Extract in the appropriate direction following the angle of the follicles to release sebum. Lancets are disposed of in biohazard containers. Remember to check with your regulatory agency to see if lancets are permitted in your area.

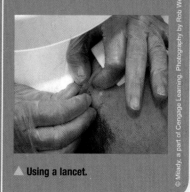

▲ **Using a lancet.**

Rubrics are used in education for organizing and interpreting data gathered from observations of student performance. It is a clearly developed scoring document used to differentiate between levels of development in a specific skill performance or behavior. Rubrics are provided in this supplement for use as either a self-assessment tool to aid the student in behavior development or as an educator assessment tool to determine competence. Space is provided to record steps needed for further growth and improvement.

Performance is evaluated according to the following scale:

1 **Development Opportunity:** There is little or no evidence of competency; assistance is needed; performance includes multiple errors.

2 **Fundamental:** There is beginning evidence of competency; task is completed alone; performance includes few errors.

3 **Competent:** There is detailed and consistent evidence of competency; task is completed alone; performance includes rare errors.

4 **Strength:** There is detailed evidence of highly creative, inventive, mature presence of competency.

Space is provided for comments to assist you in improving your performance and achieving a higher rating.

Extractions Assessment

PERFORMANCE ASSESSED	1	2	3	4	IMPROVEMENT PLAN
1. If using premade pads, applied astringent to pads and wrapped around fingers.					
2. In the absence of premade pads, dipped strips of clean cotton in water and removed excess.					
3. Unfolded pad and divided in half.					
4. Placed one-half of pad back in bowl holding pads.					
5. Lightly saturated half of pad being held with astringent.					
6. Squeezed out excess astringent.					
7. Tore small strips from the astringent-saturated cotton.					
8. Wrapped gloved index fingers with dampened pads.					
Procedure					
1. Prepared client's skin.					
2. On flat chin area, pressed down, under, and up.					
3. Worked around plug, pressing down, in, and up.					
4. Brought fingers in toward each other around the follicle without pinching.					
5. Slid fingers down each side of nose, firmly holding nostril tissue.					
6. Did not press down too firmly.					
7. Slid fingers down the cheek area, holding skin taut.					

PERFORMANCE ASSESSED	1	2	3	4	IMPROVEMENT PLAN
8. Used same technique as on chin area for forehead and upper cheekbones.					
9. Completed standard post-service procedure unless continuing with a facial treatment.					
10. Disposd of gloves and supplies properly. Changed gloves if continuing on to the facial treatment.					

Notes

_____

_____

_____

_____

_____

_____

_____

_____

_____

_____

_____

_____

_____

_____

_____

_____

_____

_____

15-8

Applying the Paraffin Mask

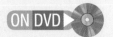
ON DVD ▶

Equipment
• Paraffin wax and heater

Supplies
• Disinfectant
• Hand sanitizer/antibacterial soap
• Paraffin wax brush
• Covered waste container
• Plastic bag
• Bowl
• Spatula
• Bolster

Linens
• Hand towels
• Client wrap
• Sheets or other linens
• Blanket
• Headband

Single-use Items
• Gauze
• Paper towels
• Gloves
• Cotton pads
• Cotton rounds
• Tissues

Products
• Cleanser
• Serum
• Mask
• Toner
• Eye cream
• Moisturizer
• Sunscreen
• Lip balm

Note: Paraffin wax masks are not used much anymore, but it is helpful to be familiar with them and they are interesting to try. It is still popular for the hands and feet.

Service Tip

• The paraffin mask can be applied in a facial or alone.
• Unscented white paraffin should be used for the face.
• Serums and ampoules used under the mask are designed for specific skin conditions.
• Gauze is used to keep paraffin and gypsum/plaster masks from sticking to the skin and the tiny hairs on the face.

Preparation

• **Perform** 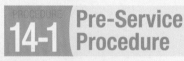 **14-1 Pre-Service Procedure** PAGE 16

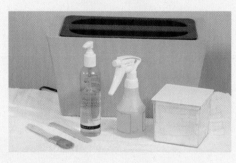

• Melt the paraffin in a warming unit to a little more than body temperature (98.6 degrees Fahrenheit or 37 degrees Celsius). The wax may take up to an hour to heat to the proper temperature.

Procedure

1 After draping and cleansing, place eye pads on client.

2 Apply an appropriate product, such as a serum or hydrating mask, under the paraffin mask.

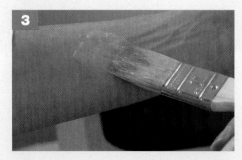
3

3 Test the temperature of the paraffin by applying to the inside of the wrist with a spatula. Discard any used wax in a plastic bag for waste disposal.

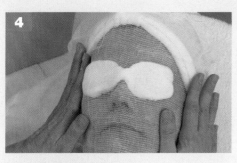

4 Cut the gauze to the desired size, and place it over the face and neck. It is not usually necessary to cut holes for the eyes and nose, because the gauze is woven very loosely. Occasionally, however, a client may feel claustrophobic. In that case, make slits in the gauze for the eyes, nose, and mouth before use. Precut gauze pads are available and are more efficient for this use.

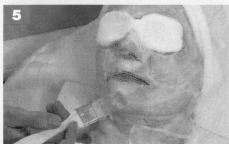

5 Apply the first coat of paraffin over the gauze with a brush, beginning at the base of the neck and working up to the forehead. Do not get wax in the hair as it is difficult to get out. Use a new spatula or brush for each layer to avoid contamination by double-dipping.

6 Continue adding layers of paraffin to the top of the gauze until the application is approximately ¼-inch (.6 centimeters) thick. The application of wax will take approximately 10 minutes.

7 After the wax application is completed, have the client relax until the wax is hardened and ready to remove (approximately 15 minutes).

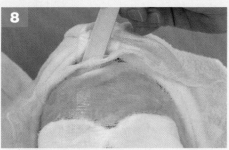

8 When ready to remove the mask, use a wooden spatula to work the edges of the mask loose from the face and neck.

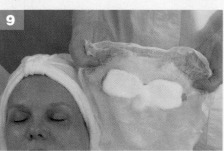

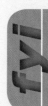

9 Carefully lift the mask from the neck in one piece.

A nice add-on service is a hand massage and paraffin dip for the hands.

10 Finish the service with the appropriate products (toner, moisturizer).

Post-Service

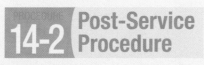

• **Complete** **14-2** **Post-Service Procedure** PAGE 22

Here's a **Tip**

To avoid double-dipping in the paraffin, put a small amount in a separate bowl and work out of that bowl with a brush. Work quickly as paraffin cools rapidly. After the service, the bowl and brush can be cleaned out and disinfected after the paraffin hardens and is removed from the bowl and brush.

Rubrics are used in education for organizing and interpreting data gathered from observations of student performance. It is a clearly developed scoring document used to differentiate between levels of development in a specific skill performance or behavior. Rubrics are provided in this supplement for use as either a self-assessment tool to aid the student in behavior development or as an educator assessment tool to determine competence. Space is provided to record steps needed for further growth and improvement.

Performance is evaluated according to the following scale:

1 **Development Opportunity:** There is little or no evidence of competency; assistance is needed; performance includes multiple errors.

2 **Fundamental:** There is beginning evidence of competency; task is completed alone; performance includes few errors.

3 **Competent:** There is detailed and consistent evidence of competency; task is completed alone; performance includes rare errors.

4 **Strength:** There is detailed evidence of highly creative, inventive, mature presence of competency.

Space is provided for comments to assist you in improving your performance and achieving a higher rating.

Applying the Paraffin Mask Assessment

PERFORMANCE ASSESSED	1	2	3	4	IMPROVEMENT PLAN
Preparation					
Completed standard pre-service procedure.					
Procedure					
1. Placed eye pads on client.					
2. Applied appropriate product (serum or hydrating mask).					
3. Tested temperature of paraffin on wrist.					
4. Cut gauze to desired size.					
5. Placed gauze over face and neck.					
6. Applied first coat of paraffin over gauze with brush.					
7. Began at neck and worked toward forehead.					
8. Continued adding paraffin until approximately ¼" (6 cm) thick.					
9. Allowed wax to harden for approximately 10–15 minutes.					
10. Used wooden spatula to work edges of mask loose from face and neck.					
11. Carefully lifted mask from neck in one piece.					
12. Completed the service with the appropriate products (toner, moisturizer).					
13. Completed standard post-service procedure unless continuing with another service.					

Notes

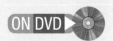

PROCEDURE
16-1

IMPLEMENTS AND MATERIALS

- Client intake form
- Disinfectant
- Hand towels
- Soap
- Covered waste container
- Bowls
- Spatulas
- Fan brush
- Bolster
- Clean linens
- Blanket
- Headband
- Client gown or wrap

Single-use Items

- Paper towels
- Cotton swabs
- Gloves/finger cots
- Cotton pads/4" × 4" pads (10 cm × 10 cm)
- Tissues
- Cotton rounds
- Plastic bag (for waste disposal)

Products

- Cleanser
- Massage lotion
- Toner
- Moisturizer
- Sunscreen for daytime
- Additional facial products if performing an entire facial

Equipment

- Facial bed/table
- Towel warmer as needed

The Facial Massage

Preparation

- **Perform** **14-1** PROCEDURE **Pre-Service Procedure** PAGE 16

It is recommended that you first practice the facial massage steps on a mannequin and write out the massage steps on an index card before doing the massage. By this point in your studies you will already have experience with the set up procedures, client consultation, and decontamination procedures.

Procedure

The following procedure is a standard relaxing massage.

- Use a product that will easily glide across the skin. Warm the product before applying.
- Start out with a light touch, gradually using firmer pressure where applicable.
- A good rule of thumb is to repeat each of the movements (each pass) consecutively three to six times.
- The number of movements to perform for each step may vary—these are only suggestions.
- Each instructor may have developed her own routine. Follow your instructor's lead.

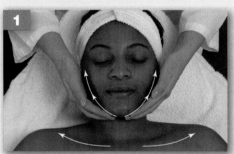

1 With clean, warm hands, evenly apply the warmed massage product to the décolleté, neck, and face by using the hands or a soft brush. One teaspoon (5 milliliters) should be enough product for the facial area.

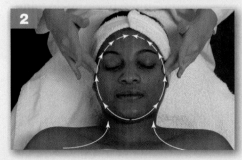

2 Start with hands on the décolleté. Move slowly up the sides of the neck and face to the forehead. Slide to each of the next steps without breaking contact or lifting fingers off the face.

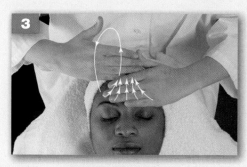

3   With the middle and ring fingers of each hand, start upward strokes in the middle of the forehead at the brow line. Working upward toward the hairline, one hand follows the other as the hands move over toward the right temple, then move back across the forehead to the left temple, and then move back to the center of the forehead. Repeat the movements three to six times.

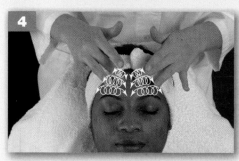

4   With the middle or index finger of each hand, start a circular movement in the middle of the forehead along the brow line. Continue this circular movement while working toward the temples. Bring the fingers back to the center of the forehead at a point between the brow line and the hairline. Move up on the forehead towards the hairline for the final movements. Each time the fingers reach the temple, pause for a moment and apply slight pressure to the temple. Repeat three to six times.

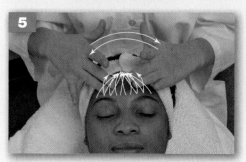

5   With the middle and ring fingers of each hand, start a crisscross stroking movement at the middle of the forehead, starting at the brow line and moving upward toward the hairline. Move toward the right temple and back to the center of the forehead. Now move toward the left temple and back to the center of the forehead. Repeat three to six times.

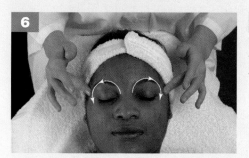

6   Place the ring fingers under the inside corners of the eyebrows and the middle fingers over the brows. Slide the fingers to the outer corner of the eye, lifting the brow at the same time. This movement continues with the next step.

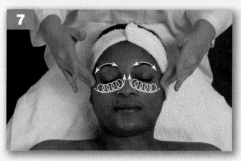

7   Start a circular movement with the middle finger at the outside corner of the eye. Continue the circular movement on the cheekbone to the point under the center of the eye, and then slide the fingers back to the starting point. Repeat six to eight times. The left hand moves clockwise, and the right hand moves counterclockwise.

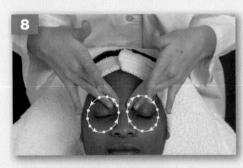

8 Start a light tapping movement with the pads of the fingers. Tap lightly around the eyes as if playing a piano. Continue tapping, moving from the temple, under the eye, toward the nose, up and over the brow, and outward to the temple. Do not tap the eyelids directly over the eyeball. Repeat six times.

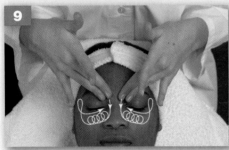

9 With the middle or index finger of each hand, start a circular movement down the nose and continuing across the cheeks to the temples. Slide the fingers under the eyes and back to the bridge of the nose. Repeat the movements six times.

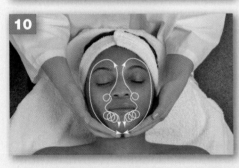

10 With the middle and ring fingers of each hand, slide the fingers from the bridge of the nose, over the brow (lifting the brow), and down to the chin. Start a firm circular movement on the chin with the thumbs. Change to the middle fingers at the corner of the mouth. Rotate the fingers five times, and slide the fingers up the sides of the nose, over the brow, and then stop for a moment at the temple. Apply slight pressure on the temple. Slide the fingers down to the chin, and repeat the movements six times. The downward movement on the side of the face should have a very light touch to avoid dragging the skin downward.

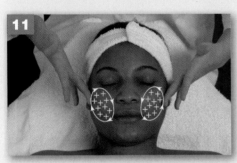

11 With the pads of the fingertips, start a light tapping movement (piano playing) on the cheeks, working in a circle around the cheeks. Repeat the movements six to eight times.

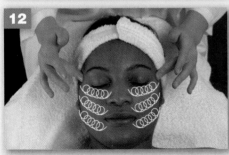

12 Slide to the center of the chin. Using a finger of each hand, start a circular movement at the center of the chin and move up to the earlobes. Slide the middle fingers to the corner of the mouth and then continue the circular movements to the middle of the ears. Return the middle fingers to the nose and continue the circular movements outward across the cheeks to the top of the ear. Repeat each of the three passes three to six times. Slide down to the mouth.

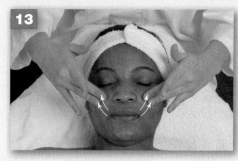

13 Place one finger above the mouth and one finger below the mouth. With the index and middle fingers of each hand, start the "scissor" movement, gliding from the center of the mouth, upward over the cheekbone, and stopping at the top of the cheekbone. Alternate the movement from one side of the face to the other, using the right hand on the right side of the face and then the left hand on the left side. As one hand reaches the cheekbone, start the other at the center of the mouth. Repeat eight to ten times.

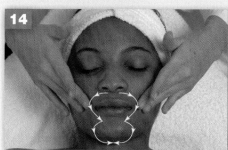

14 With the middle finger of both hands, draw the fingers from the center of the upper lip, around the mouth, under the lower lip, and then continue a circle under the chin. Repeat six to eight times.

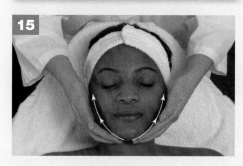

15 With the index finger above the chin and jawline (the middle, ring, and little fingers should be under the chin and jaw), start a scissor movement from the center of the chin and then slide the fingers along the jawline to the earlobe. Alternate one hand after the other, using the right hand on the right side of the face and the left hand on the left side of the face. Repeat eight to ten times on each side of the face. Slide down to the neck.

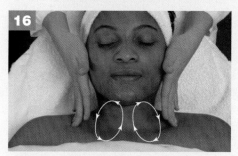

16 Apply light upward strokes over the front of the neck with both hands. Circle down and then back up, using firmer downward pressure on the outer sides of the neck. Repeat 10 times. Do not press down on the center of the neck.

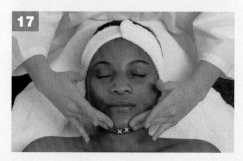

17 With the middle and ring fingers of the right hand, give two quick taps under the chin, followed with one quick tap with the middle and ring fingers of the left hand. The taps should be done in a continuous movement, keeping a steady rhythm. The taps should be done with a light touch, but with enough pressure so that a soft tapping sound can be heard. Continue the tapping movement while moving the hands slightly to the right and then to the left, so as to cover the complete underside of the chin. Without stopping or breaking the rhythm of the tapping, move to the right cheek.

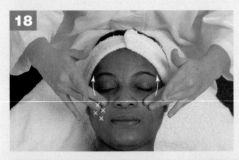

18 Continue the tapping on the right cheek in the same manner as under the chin, except the tapping with the left hand will have a lifting movement. The rhythm will be tap, tap, lift, tap, tap, lift, tap, tap, lift. Repeat this rhythmic movement 15 to 20 times. Without stopping the tapping movement, move the fingers back under the chin and over the left cheek, repeating the tapping and lifting movements. Move up and out on the area in a consistent pattern. Avoid tapping directly on the jawbone because this will feel unpleasant to the client.

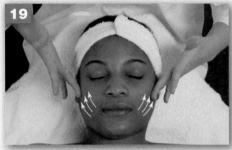

19 Without stopping the tapping movement, move the hands over to the corners of the mouth. Break into an upward, stroking movement with the first three fingers of each hand. One finger follows the other as each finger lifts the corner of the mouth. Use both hands at the same time or alternate each hand—as one hand ends the movement, the other starts. Repeat the stroking movement 15 to 20 times.

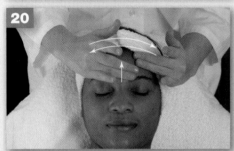

20 Without stopping the stroking movement, move up to the outside corner of the left eye and continue the stroking, upward movement. Continue the stoking movement across the forehead to the outside corner of the right eye. Continue this stroking movement back and forth 10 times in each direction.

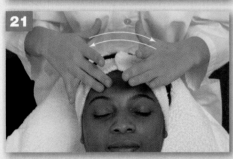

21 Continue the stroking movement back and forth across the forehead, gradually slowing the movement. Let the movements grow slower and slower as the touch becomes lighter and lighter. Taper the movement off until the fingers are gradually lifted from the forehead. This slowing down of movement is often called *feathering*.

Optional: Glide down to the neck and chest and repeat the movements on these areas as directed by your instructor.

22 Finish the facial service, and complete your client consultation.

Post-Service

• **Complete** **PROCEDURE 14-2** **Post-Service Procedure** PAGE 22

fyi

Blood returning to the heart from the head, face, and neck flows down the jugular veins on each side of the neck. All massage movements on the side of the neck are done with a downward (never upward) motion. Always slide gently upward in the center of the neck and circle out and then down on the sides. This also assists with fluid and lymph drainage.

Rubrics are used in education for organizing and interpreting data gathered from observations of student performance. It is a clearly developed scoring document used to differentiate between levels of development in a specific skill performance or behavior. Rubrics are provided in this supplement for use as either a self-assessment tool to aid the student in behavior development or as an educator assessment tool to determine competence. Space is provided to record steps needed for further growth and improvement.

Performance is evaluated according to the following scale:

1 Development Opportunity: There is little or no evidence of competency; assistance is needed; Performance includes multiple errors.

2 Fundamental: There is beginning evidence of competency; task is completed alone; performance includes few errors.

3 Competent: There is detailed and consistent evidence of competency; task is completed alone; performance includes rare errors.

4 Strength: There is detailed evidence of highly creative, inventive, mature presence of competency.

Space is provided for comments to assist you in improving your performance and achieving a higher rating.

The Facial Massage Assessment

PERFORMANCE ASSESSED	1	2	3	4	IMPROVEMENT PLAN
Preparation					
Completed standard pre-service procedure.					
Procedure					
1. Cleansed own hands.					
2. Applied warm massage product to décolleté and face.					
3. Started at décolleté and moved slowly up sides of neck and face to the forehead.					
4. With middle and forefingers of both hands, applied upward strokes at the center of the forehead moving to the outside temples and back to center.					
5. Repeated forehead movement 3 to 6 times.					
6. Applied circular movement with middle finger along the brow line and worked toward temples.					
7. Paused at the temples.					
8. Repeated 3 to 6 times.					
9. With middle and ring fingers, performed the crisscross stroking movement on forehead.					
10. Repeated crisscross movement 3 to 6 times.					
11. Slid ring and middle fingers over brows to the outer corner of the eye, lifting brow at the same time.					
12. Performed circular movement, using middle fingers, from the outside corner of the eye to under the center of the eye.					

PERFORMANCE ASSESSED	1	2	3	4	IMPROVEMENT PLAN
13. Repeated movement 6 to 8 times.					
14. Performed a light tapping movement around the eyes, moving from temples to under the eyes, toward the nose, up and over the brow, and outward to the temple.					
15. Repeated movement 6 times.					
16. Began a circular movement down the nose and continued across the cheeks to the temples.					
17. Slid fingers under the eyes and back to bridge of nose.					
18. Repeated movements 6 times.					
19. Slid fingers from bridge of nose, over brow while lifting, and down to the chin.					
20. Began a firm circular movement on the chin with thumbs.					
21. Changed to middle fingers at corner of mouth.					
22. Rotated fingers 5 times.					
23. Slid fingers up sides of nose, over brow, paused at temple and applied pressure.					
24. Slid fingers down to chin.					
25. Repeated movement 6 times.					
26. Performed a light tapping movement on the cheeks, working in a circle around the cheeks.					
27. Repeated movement 6 to 8 times.					
28. Began circular movement at center of chin and moved up to earlobes.					
29. Slid middle fingers to corner of mouth and continued circular movements to middle of ears.					
30. Returned middle fingers to nose and continued circular movements outward across cheeks to the top of ear.					
31. Repeat each pass 3 to 6 times.					
32. Slid down to mouth.					
33. Performed the "scissor" movement from center of mouth to top of cheekbones.					
34. Alternated "scissor" movement from one side of face to the other.					
35. Repeated movement 8 to 10 times.					
36. Drew fingers from center of upper lip, around mouth, under lower lip, and under chin.					

PERFORMANCE ASSESSED	1	2	3	4	IMPROVEMENT PLAN
37. Repeated movement 6 to 8 times.					
38. Began a "scissor" movement at center of chin.					
39. Slid fingers along jawline to the earlobe.					
40. Repeated 8 to 10 times on each side of face.					
41. With both hands, applied light upward strokes over front of neck.					
42. Circled down and then back up, using firmer downward pressure on the outer sides of neck.					
43. Repeated movement 10 times.					
44. Performed the tapping movement under chin keeping a steady rhythm.					
45. Continued tapping to lift chin area and moved to right cheek.					
46. Repeated rhythmic movement 15 to 20 times.					
47. Avoided tapping directly on the jawbone.					
48. Performed a stroking movement at the mouth.					
49. Repeated movement 15 to 20 times.					
50. Moved up to the outside corner of left eye and across forehead to outside corner of the right eye.					
51. Repeated stroking movement 10 times in each direction.					
52. Continued stroking movement across forehead.					
53. Gradually slowed movements.					
54. Feathered off at end of massage.					
Post-Service					
Completed standard post-service, cleanup, and disinfection procedures or proceeded to next service (such as completing a facial).					

IMPLEMENTS AND MATERIALS

- Station and cleaning supplies
- EPA-registered disinfectant
- Hand sanitizer
- Towels
- Tweezers
- Small hair scissors
- Small hand-held mirror
- Cotton pads
- Eyebrow brush or comb
- Emollient cream
- Antiseptic lotion
- Gentle eye makeup remover
- Astringent
- Single-use gloves
- Client release form and chart
- Client headband
- Plastic bag for disposables

Eyebrow Tweezing

Preparation

- **Perform** 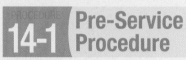 **14-1 Pre-Service Procedure** PAGE 16

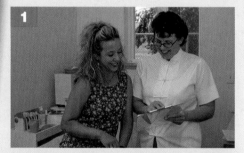

1 Discuss with the client the type of eyebrow arch suitable for her facial characteristics.

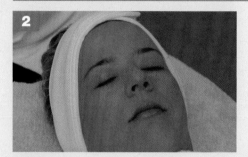

2 Seat the client in a facial chair in a reclining position, as for a facial massage. Or, if you prefer, seat the client in a half-upright position and work from the side if it is comfortable for both you and the client. The head needs to be supported and held steady to get a firm grip and hold the skin taut. The brows should be easy to reach and visible under adequate lighting, preferably with a magnifying light.

3 Drape a towel over the client's clothing.

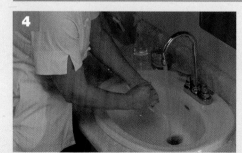

4 Wash and dry your hands, and put on single-use gloves. Washing your hands thoroughly with soap and warm water is critical before and after every client procedure you perform. The importance of proper cleaning in these procedures cannot be overemphasized.

Procedure

The eyebrow tweezing procedure involves the following steps:

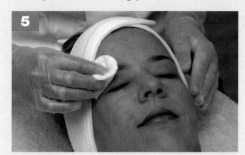

5 Prepare the skin: use a mild antiseptic on a cotton pad before tweezing to clean and prepare the area.

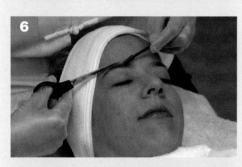

6 Measure the brows to check the shape (in-between the brows, the arch, and the end of the brow). Brush the eyebrows with a small brush. Carefully trim long hairs outside the brow line now or after tweezing. Brush the hair upward and into place to see the natural line of the brow. Observe the stray hairs and what needs to be removed.

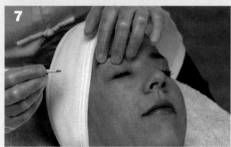

7 Stretch the skin taut next to the hair with the index finger and thumb (or index and middle fingers) of your other hand while tweezing. Hold each area taut next to the hair being removed.

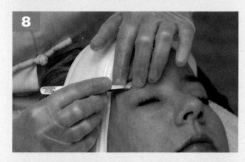

8 Remove hairs from under the eyebrow line. Shape the lower section of one eyebrow, then shape the other. Grasp each hair individually with tweezers and pull with a quick, smooth motion in the direction of the hair growth. Carefully grasp the hair at the base as close to the skin as possible without pinching the skin and pull in the direction of the hair growth, not straight up or out.

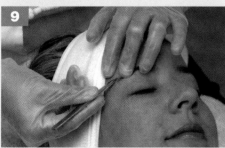

9 Brush the hair downward. Remove hairs from above the eyebrow line if the predetermined shape deems it neccessary. Shape the upper section of one eyebrow; then shape the other.

18-1

18-1 Eyebrow Tweezing (continued)

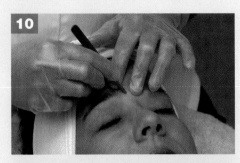

10 Remove hair from between the brows.

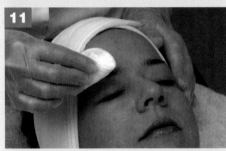

11 Wipe the tweezed areas with a cotton pad, moistened with a nonirritating antiseptic lotion, to contract the skin and avoid infection.

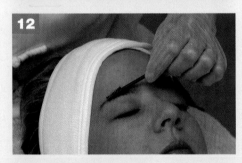

12 Brush the eyebrow hair in its normal position.

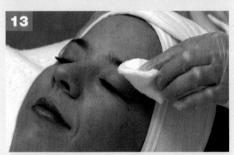

13 *Optional:* Apply a soothing cream. Gently remove excess cream with a cotton pad.

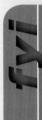

fyi

Always wash your hands before preparing and setting up for a service, after draping, immediately after any service before walking the client out, and after finishing the post-service procedures.

14 If eyebrow tweezing is part of a makeup or facial service, continue the procedure. If not, complete the next step.

Post-Service

• Complete **14-2** Post-Service Procedure PAGE 22

Rubrics are used in education for organizing and interpreting data gathered from observations of student performance. It is a clearly developed scoring document used to differentiate between levels of development in a specific skill performance or behavior. Rubrics are provided in this supplement for use as either a self-assessment tool to aid the student in behavior development or as an educator assessment tool to determine competence. Space is provided to record steps needed for further growth and improvement.

Performance is evaluated according to the following scale:

1   **Development Opportunity:** There is little or no evidence of competency; assistance is needed; performance includes multiple errors.

2   **Fundamental:** There is beginning evidence of competency; task is completed alone; performance includes few errors.

3   **Competent:** There is detailed and consistent evidence of competency; task is completed alone; performance includes rare errors.

4   **Strength:** There is detailed evidence of highly creative, inventive, mature presence of competency.

Space is provided for comments to assist you in improving your performance and achieving a higher rating.

18-1

Eyebrow Tweezing Assessment

PERFORMANCE ASSESSED	1	2	3	4	IMPROVEMENT PLAN
Preparation					
1. Completed standard pre-service procedure.					
2. Discussed the suitable arch for the client's facial characteristics.					
3. Helped client prepare for the service.					
4. Properly placed headband.					
5. Draped towel over client's clothing.					
6. Washed and dried own hands.					
7. Put on disposable gloves.					
Procedure					
1. Prepared area by applying a mild antiseptic with a cotton pad.					
2. Measured brows to check shape.					
3. Brushed eyebrows with brow brush.					
4. Carefully trimmed long hairs outside brow line.					
5. Stretched the skin taut with index finger and thumb.					
6. Removed hairs from under the brow line.					
7. Shaped lower section of one eyebrow, then the other.					
8. Grasped individual hair with tweezers and pulled with a quick, smooth motion in the direction of hair growth.					
9. Brushed brow hairs downward.					

PERFORMANCE ASSESSED	1	2	3	4	IMPROVEMENT PLAN
10. Shaped upper section of one brow, then the other.					
11. Removed hair from between brows.					
12. Sponged tweezed areas with a cotton pad moistened with antiseptic lotion.					
13. Brushed eyebrow hair into normal placement.					
14. Optional: Applied a smoothing cream to area.					
15. Removed excess cream with a cotton pad.					
16. Proceeded with additional services as applicable.					
Post-Service					
Completed standard post-service, cleanup, and disinfection procedures.					

Notes

_____

_____

_____

_____

_____

_____

_____

_____

_____

_____

_____

_____

_____

Eyebrow Waxing with Soft Wax

IMPLEMENTS AND MATERIALS

The following list applies for all waxing procedures.

- Facial chair or treatment table
- Technician stool
- EPA-registered disinfectant
- Hand sanitizer
- Roll of single-use paper or paper towels
- Closed, covered waste container
- Cart
- Implement tray
- Containers for supplies
- Wax product
- Wax heater
- Wax remover
- Small single-use applicators (brow size spatulas)
- Wax strips (for soft wax)
- Single-use gloves
- Sealable plastic bags for waste disposal
- Cotton pads and swabs
- Powder
- Mild skin cleanser
- Emollient or antiseptic lotion
- Brow brush
- Tweezers
- Small scissors
- Hand mirror
- Tongs (to retrieve clean supplies during a service)
- Surface cleaner (oil to remove wax from the equipment)
- Wax cleaning towels/supplies
- Table linens/towels
- Hair cap or headband for face waxing
- Towels for draping
- Wax release form and client chart
- Biohazard container, especially for underarm, bikini, and back waxing (the potenial for blood spots from follicles is normal)

This procedure for eyebrow waxing employs the use of a strip to remove soft wax. Hard wax may also be used. Adapt this procedure and supply list for all other body areas to be waxed. Review the wax application and removal techniques in the chapter before performing this procedure.

Preparation

- **Perform** **PROCEDURE 14-1** **Pre-Service Procedure** PAGE 16

- For the waxing procedures, melt the wax in the heater. The length of time it takes to melt the wax depends on the product, temperature, and how full the wax holder is: approximately 30 minutes if it is full; 15 minutes if it is a quarter to half full. Be sure the wax is not too hot.

- Complete the client consultation, release form, determine any contraindications, and determine what hair you need to remove.

- Lay a clean towel over the top of the facial chair and then a layer of single-use paper under the head (if applicable).

Procedure

The soft pot wax procedure with strips includes the following steps:

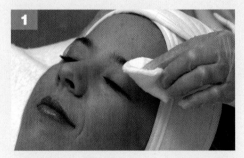

1 Prepare the skin: remove makeup on the area to be waxed. Cleanse the area thoroughly with a mild astringent cleanser, and dry.

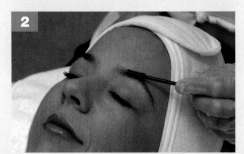

2 Apply a non-talc powder, if applicable. Brush the hair into place to see the brow line. Measure the three lines for shaping and examine what hair needs to be removed.

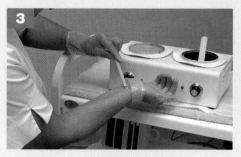

3 Test the temperature and consistency of the heated wax by applying a small (dime size) drop on the inside of your wrist. It should be warm but not hot, and it should run smoothly off the spatula. Remove with a strip as you would while waxing.

4 Wipe off one side of the spatula on the inside edge of the pot, so it does not drip. Carefully take it from the pot to the brow area. If it is dripping off the spatula, there is too much wax, or it is too hot. Correct the problem to avoid drips or hurting the client.

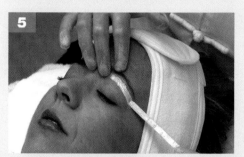

5 Apply the wax: with the spatula at a 45-degree angle, spread a thin coat of the wax evenly over the area to be waxed, following the direction of the hair growth. Hold the skin taut near the edge where the wax is first applied. Be sure not to put the spatula in the wax more than once (do not double-dip). Do not use an excessive amount of wax, because it will spread when the fabric is pressed and may cover hair you do not wish to remove.

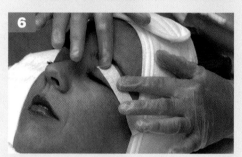

6 Apply a clean fabric strip over the area to be waxed. Start the edge of the strip at the edge of the wax where you first applied it. Do not cover the rest of the brow with the strip. This way you can see the exposed area that you do not want to wax. Leave enough of the strip to hold on to for the pull. Press gently in the direction of hair growth, running your finger over the surface of the fabric three to five times so the wax adheres to the hair. Remember to check to make sure wax has not spread where you do not want it.

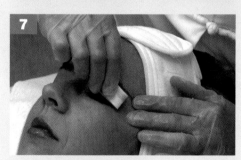

7 Remove the wax: gently but firmly hold the skin taut, placing the index and middle fingers of one hand on next to the strip as close as possible to where you will start to pull. Hold the loose edge of the strip at the end and quickly remove the strip by pulling in the direction opposite to the hair growth. Do not lift or pull straight up on the strip; doing so could damage or remove the skin.

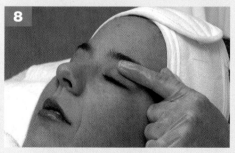

8 Immediately apply pressure with your finger to the waxed area. Hold it there for approximately 5 seconds to relieve the painful sensation.

9 Remove any excess wax residue from the skin with the strip by gently lifting it sideways in the same direction as the hair growth. To avoid removing additional hair, do not let the strip accidently touch any hair while doing this. A clean part of the strip can be folded over and used for this, or use a new strip.

10 Repeat the wax procedure on the area around the other eyebrow.

18-2

18-2 Eyebrow Waxing with Soft Wax (continued)

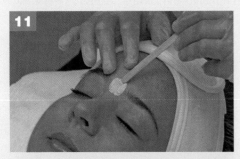

11 For the area between the brows, apply the wax (generally in an upward direction between the nose and the forehead). Line the bottom of the strip up to the bottom edge of the wax. Hold the skin taut on both sides of the strip above the brows with the middle and ring fingers.

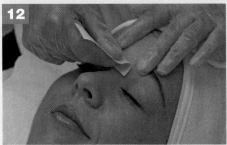

12 Hold the top of the strip and pull the strip straight down close to the nose without lifting. This area can be done all in one section or in two halves—the right and the left.

> **CAUTION!**
>
> Never leave the wax heater on overnight, because it is a fire hazard and can affect the quality of the wax.

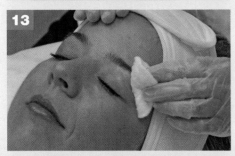

13 Cleanse the waxed area with a mild wax-remover, and apply a post-wax product or antiseptic lotion.

> **Service Tip**
>
> Excess wax will get on the tweezers and interfere with tweezing. Remove all wax and post-products with a moist cotton pad before tweezing, and reapply soothing products after tweezing.

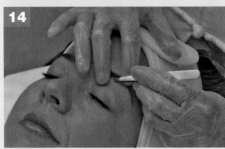

14 Tweeze the remaining stray hairs, and apply a cold compress if necessary. If it is too slippery or there is wax residue, apply the post-wax products after tweezing or rinse the area with water and pat dry before tweezing.

15 Remove the gloves and wash your hands.

Post-Service

- **Complete** **PROCEDURE 14-2 Post-Service Procedure** PAGE 22

- Discard all used single-use materials in a sealable plastic bag and closed waste container.
- Never reuse wax.
- Do not place the used spatula, muslin strips, wax, or any other materials used in waxing directly on the counter. Use a tray or paper towel.
- Complete a post-wax consultation and discuss post-wax precautions.

> **CAUTION!**
>
> If the wax strings and lands in an area you do not wish to treat, remove it with lotion designed to dissolve and remove wax. Always cover clients' hair and clothes to protect them from wax.

Rubrics are used in education for organizing and interpreting data gathered from observations of student performance. It is a clearly developed scoring document used to differentiate between levels of development in a specific skill performance or behavior. Rubrics are provided in this supplement for use as either a self-assessment tool to aid the student in behavior development or as an educator assessment tool to determine competence. Space is provided to record steps needed for further growth and improvement.

Performance is evaluated according to the following scale:

1 **Development Opportunity:** There is little or no evidence of competency; assistance is needed; performance includes multiple errors.

2 **Fundamental:** There is beginning evidence of competency; task is completed alone; performance includes few errors.

3 **Competent:** There is detailed and consistent evidence of competency; task is completed alone; performance includes rare errors.

4 **Strength:** There is detailed evidence of highly creative, inventive, mature presence of competency.

Space is provided for comments to assist you in improving your performance and achieving a higher rating.

Eyebrow Waxing with Soft Wax Assessment

PERFORMANCE ASSESSED	1	2	3	4	IMPROVEMENT PLAN
Preparation					
1. Completed standard pre-service procedure.					
2. Melted wax in heater for approximately 10 to 20 minutes.					
3. Properly placed headband.					
4. Draped towel over top of facial chair.					
5. Placed layer of single-use paper under head.					
6. Washed and dried own hands.					
7. Put on disposable gloves.					
Procedure					
1. Prepared area by cleansing with a mild antiseptic on a cotton pad.					
2. Dried area thoroughly.					
3. Applied a non-talc powder.					
4. Brushed hair into place to see brow line.					
5. Tested temperature and consistency of wax.					
6. Dipped spatula in wax.					
7. Took appropriate steps to prevent dripping.					
8. Spread a thin coat of warm wax over area to be treated following hair growth (did not double-dip).					
9. Held skin taut near edge where wax was first applied.					

PERFORMANCE ASSESSED	1	2	3	4	IMPROVEMENT PLAN
10. Applied fabric strip over area to be waxed.					
11. Did not cover rest of brow with strip.					
12. Pressed gently in direction of hair growth, running fingers over surface multiple times.					
13. Gently, but firmly, held the skin taut and quickly removed the fabric strip.					
14. Pulled the fabric strip in the direction opposite to hair growth.					
15. Applied pressure with fingers to treated area.					
16. Maintained pressure for 5 seconds.					
17. Removed excess wax residue from skin with cotton strip.					
18. Repeated procedure on other eyebrow.					
19. Applied wax between brows in an upward direction between nose and forehead.					
20. Lined bottom edge of strip up with bottom edge of wax application and applied.					
21. Held skin taut and pulled strip downward in one or two steps.					
22. Cleansed skin with a mild wax remover.					
23. Applied a post-wax product or antiseptic lotion.					
24. Tweezed remaining stray hairs.					
25. Removed gloves.					
Post-Service					
Completed standard post-service, cleanup, and disinfection procedures.					

Notes

18-3

Lip Waxing with Hard Wax

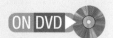
ON DVD ►

IMPLEMENTS AND MATERIALS

- Facial chair or treatment table
- Technician stool
- EPA-registered disinfectant
- Hand sanitizer
- Roll of single-use paper or paper towels
- Closed, covered waste container
- Cart
- Implement tray
- Containers for supplies
- Wax product
- Wax heater
- Wax remover
- Single-use applicators (medium size spatulas)
- Wax strips (for soft wax)
- Single-use gloves
- Sealable plastic bags for waste disposal
- Cotton pads and swabs
- Powder
- Mild skin cleanser
- Emollient or antiseptic lotion
- Tweezers
- Small scissors
- Hand mirror
- Tongs (to retrieve clean supplies during a service)
- Surface cleaner (oil to remove wax from the equipment)
- Wax cleaning towels/supplies
- Table linens/towels
- Hair cap or headband for face waxing
- Towels for draping
- Wax release form and client chart
- Biohazard container, especially for underarm, bikini, and back waxing (the potenial for blood spots from follicles is normal)

Be guided by your instructor for hard wax application and removal. Some apply and remove hard wax differently than soft wax. For example: Only with hard wax can you apply opposite to the hair growth and remove with the direction of the hair growth. It is best to learn the soft wax techniques first to avoid incorrect pulls and injuring the skin.

Preparation

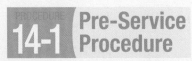

- **Perform** **14-1** **Pre-Service Procedure** PAGE 16

- Melt the wax in the heater.

Note: Soft wax may be used with strips for the same procedure. The lip waxing procedure with hard wax includes the following steps:

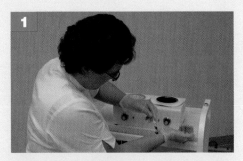

1 After draping the client, test the temperature and consistency of the wax on the inside of your wrist.

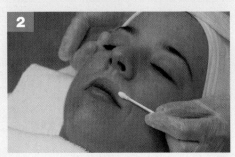

2 Prepare the skin by cleansing. For lip waxing, have the client hold the lips tightly together to avoid pulling the skin.

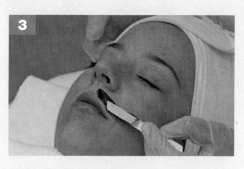

3 Apply wax to one side of the upper lip outward from the center to the corner, leaving a "tab" or "handle" to grasp. Make sure there is a thicker layer of hard wax and the consistency is right before removing. It should be firm and feel tacky, but not hard or brittle. (If using soft wax, apply the strip.)

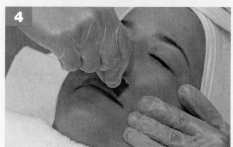

4 Remove the wax: hold the skin taut, and quickly pull parallel to the skin without lifting up.

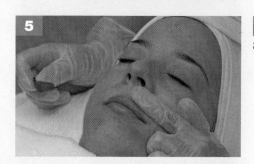

5 Immediately apply pressure to the waxed area to ease any discomfort.

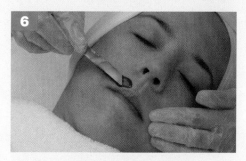

6 Repeat on the other side of the lip.

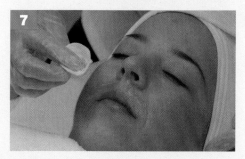

7 Apply after-wax soothing lotion.

Post-Service

• **Complete** **PROCEDURE 14-2** **Post-Service Procedure** PAGE 22

• Complete a post-wax consultation and discuss post-wax precautions.

18-3

Rubrics are used in education for organizing and interpreting data gathered from observations of student performance. It is a clearly developed scoring document used to differentiate between levels of development in a specific skill performance or behavior. Rubrics are provided in this supplement for use as either a self-assessment tool to aid the student in behavior development or as an educator assessment tool to determine competence. Space is provided to record steps needed for further growth and improvement.

Performance is evaluated according to the following scale:

1 **Development Opportunity:** There is little or no evidence of competency; assistance is needed; Performance includes multiple errors.

2 **Fundamental:** There is beginning evidence of competency; task is completed alone; performance includes few errors.

3 **Competent:** There is detailed and consistent evidence of competency; task is completed alone; performance includes rare errors.

4 **Strength:** There is detailed evidence of highly creative, inventive, mature presence of competency.

Space is provided for comments to assist you in improving your performance and achieving a higher rating.

Lip Waxing with Hard Wax Assessment

PERFORMANCE ASSESSED	1	2	3	4	IMPROVEMENT PLAN
Preparation					
1. Completed standard pre-service procedure.					
2. Melted wax in heater for approximately 10 to 20 minutes.					
3. Properly draped client.					
4. Tested wax temperature.					
Procedure					
1. Prepared area and had client hold lips tightly together.					
2. Applied wax to one side of upper lip outward from center to corner					
3. Held skin taut and quickly pulled wax parallel to skin.					
4. Immediately applied pressure to waxed area to ease discomfort.					
5. Repeated procedure on other side of lip.					
6. Applied after-wax soothing lotion.					
Post-Service					
1. Completed a post-wax consultation and discussed post-wax precautions.					
2. Completed standard post-service, cleanup, and disinfection procedures.					

Notes

18-4

Chin Waxing with Hard Wax

IMPLEMENTS AND MATERIALS

Note: Make sure you have the correct strip sizes ready if you are using soft wax instead of hard wax.

The following list applies for all waxing procedures.

- Facial chair or treatment table
- Technician stool
- EPA-registered disinfectant
- Hand sanitizer
- Roll of single-use paper or paper towels
- Closed, covered waste container
- Cart
- Implement tray
- Containers for supplies
- Wax product
- Wax heater
- Wax remover
- Single-use applicators (medium size spatulas)
- Wax strips (for soft wax)
- Single-use gloves
- Sealable plastic bags for waste disposal
- Cotton pads and swabs
- Powder
- Mild skin cleanser
- Emollient or antiseptic lotion
- Tweezers
- Small scissors
- Hand mirror
- Tongs (to retrieve clean supplies during a service)
- Surface cleaner (oil to remove wax from the equipment)
- Wax cleaning towels/supplies
- Table linens/towels
- Hair cap or headband for face waxing
- Towels for draping
- Wax release form and client chart
- Biohazard container, especially for underarm, bikini, and back waxing (the potenial for blood spots from follicles is normal)

Preparation

- **Perform** **14-1** Pre-Service Procedure   PAGE 16
- Melt the wax in the heater. Be sure the wax is not too hot.
- Complete the client consultation, release form, determine any contraindications, and determine what hair you need to remove.
- Lay a clean towel over the top of the facial chair and then a layer of single-use paper under the head (if applicable).

Procedure

1 Test the wax temperature.

2
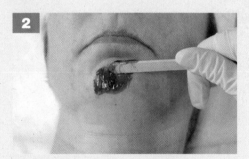

2   Apply the wax in small sections above the curve of the jawline from the top to bottom ending at the jawline. Do not go over the curve. Wax above the jawline, then below it using separate pulls. Or you can wax below the jawline first, then above it. Make sure to leave enough wax beyond the area for a handle/pull tab. Lift up the pull tab to grasp onto. Check that the wax consistency is "tacky" before removal.

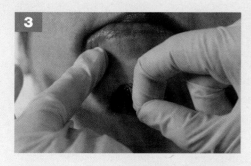

3 Remove the wax: hold the skin taut close to the end of the wax where you start the pull, and pull opposite to the hair growth and parallel to the skin.

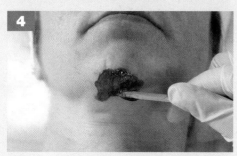

4 Apply the wax in small sections below the curve of the jawline.

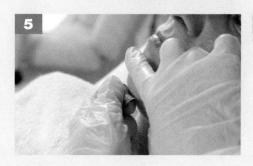

5 Remove the wax: hold the skin taut, and pull parallel to the skin.

6 Apply light pressure on the waxed area without pressing down hard on the throat or neck.

7 Continue the procedure and apply the post-wax products.

Post-Service

- **Complete** PROCEDURE **14-2** **Post-Service Procedure** PAGE 22
- Complete a post-wax consultation and discuss post-wax precautions.

18-4

Rubrics are used in education for organizing and interpreting data gathered from observations of student performance. It is a clearly developed scoring document used to differentiate between levels of development in a specific skill performance or behavior. Rubrics are provided in this supplement for use as either a self-assessment tool to aid the student in behavior development or as an educator assessment tool to determine competence. Space is provided to record steps needed for further growth and improvement.

Performance is evaluated according to the following scale:

1 **Development Opportunity:** There is little or no evidence of competency; assistance is needed; performance includes multiple errors.

2 **Fundamental:** There is beginning evidence of competency; task is completed alone; performance includes few errors.

3 **Competent:** There is detailed and consistent evidence of competency; task is completed alone; performance includes rare errors.

4 **Strength:** There is detailed evidence of highly creative, inventive, mature presence of competency.

Space is provided for comments to assist you in improving your performance and achieving a higher rating.

Chin Waxing with Hard Wax Assessment

PERFORMANCE ASSESSED	1	2	3	4	IMPROVEMENT PLAN
Preparation					
1. Completed standard pre-service procedure.					
2. Melted wax in heater for approximately 10 to 20 minutes.					
3. Placed clean towel over top of facial chair.					
4. Placed layer of single-use paper under the head.					
5. Tested wax temperature.					
Procedure					
1. Applied wax in small sections above the curve of the jawline.					
2. Left a handle/pull tab on wax strip.					
3. Held skin taut.					
4. Pulled wax opposite to hair growth and parallel to skin.					
5. Applied pressure to reduce discomfort.					
6. Applied wax in small sections below curve of jawline.					
7. Held skin tight.					
8. Pulled wax opposite to hair growth and parallel to skin.					
9. Applied pressure.					
10. Completed the procedure.					
11. Applied post-wax products.					

PERFORMANCE ASSESSED	1	2	3	4	IMPROVEMENT PLAN
Post-Service					
1. Completed a post-wax consultation and discussed post-wax precautions.					
2. Completed standard post-service, cleanup, and disinfection procedure.					

Notes

_____

_____

_____

_____

_____

_____

_____

_____

_____

_____

_____

_____

_____

_____

_____

_____

_____

_____

_____

18-4

Leg Waxing with Soft Wax

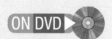
ON DVD ►

IMPLEMENTS AND MATERIALS

Note: Make sure you have the correct strip sizes ready if you are using soft wax instead of hard wax.

The following list applies for all waxing procedures.

- Facial chair or treatment table
- Technician stool
- EPA-registered disinfectant
- Hand sanitizer
- Roll of single-use paper or paper towels
- Closed, covered waste container
- Cart
- Implement tray
- Containers for supplies
- Wax product
- Wax heater
- Wax remover
- Single-use applicators (large spatulas)
- Wax strips (for soft wax)
- Single-use gloves
- Sealable plastic bags for waste disposal
- Cotton pads and swabs
- Powder
- Mild skin cleanser
- Emollient or antiseptic lotion
- Brow brush
- Tweezers
- Small scissors
- Hand mirror
- Tongs (to retrieve clean supplies during a service)
- Surface cleaner (oil to remove wax from the equipment)
- Wax cleaning towels/supplies
- Table linens/towels
- Hair cap or headband for face waxing
- Towels for draping
- Client wrap for body waxing
- Wax release form and client chart
- Biohazard container, especially for underarm, bikini, and back waxing (the potential for blood spots from follicles is normal)

Preparation

- **Perform** 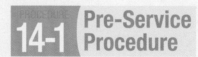 **Pre-Service Procedure** PAGE 16

- Melt the wax in the heater. Be sure the wax is not too hot.
- Complete the client consultation, release form, and determine any contraindications.
- Place a clean sheet or sheet of paper on the waxing table for each new client.

Procedure

Leg waxing can be started with either the front or the back of the legs. Visually divide the front of the legs in quarter sections (below the knees) and use a set pattern, starting removal at the bottom half of the lower legs. Make sure the skin is held taut while removing the wax, especially around the ankle, which is more sensitive.

Start the application on the front (or back) side of the leg 7 inches (17.5 centimeters) below the knee and apply down to the just above the ankle. Work across to the other side of the leg using two or three strips. Then do the next section from the middle of the lower leg to the knees. The entire front leg should be waxed, including the knees, and lotion applied to the front before having the client turn over and continue on the back of the legs.

1 If skin is moist or oily, cleanse the area to be waxed with a mild astringent cleanser and dry. If skin is dry and flaky, a tiny amount of lotion may be applied and then removed. Apply a light dusting of powder if necessary.

2 Test the temperature and consistency of the heated wax.

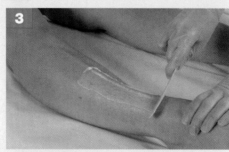

3 Apply the wax using a spatula. Spread a thin coat of warm wax evenly over the skin surface in the same direction as the hair growth.

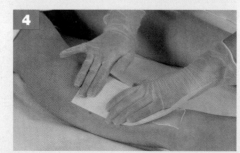

4 Apply a fabric strip over the wax in the same direction as the hair growth. Press gently but firmly, rubbing your hand back and forth over the surface of the fabric three to five times.

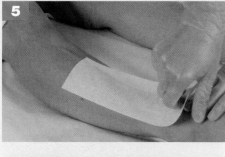

5 Remove the wax: hold the skin taut with one hand close to where you will pull with the other hand, and quickly remove the wax in the opposite direction of the hair growth without lifting.

6 Quickly put your hand down to apply pressure to the waxed area for approximately 5 seconds.

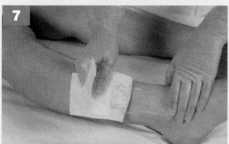

7 Repeat, using a fresh fabric strip as each strip becomes too thick with wax or hair.

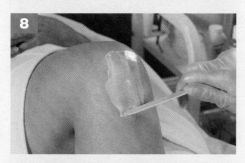

8 Wax the knees. Have the client bend the knee and place the foot on the table. Wax below the curve of the knee working in three sections across from one side to the other: left, middle, and right sides. Then wax the top of the knees above the curve using the same pattern in three sections.

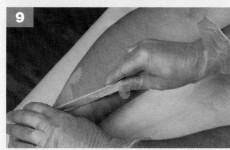

9 To keep the client's skin from sticking to the table, apply the soothing wax remover (made for the skin) only where the wax was applied before having the client turn over to wax the back of the legs. Have the client turn over, and repeat the procedure on the backs of the legs.

18-5

10 Remove any remaining residue of wax from the skin, and apply an emollient or antiseptic lotion. Check for stray hairs. Remove gloves and wash your hands after the service.

Post-Service

- **Complete** PROCEDURE **14-2** **Post-Service Procedure**   PAGE 22

- Complete a post-wax consultation and discuss post-wax precautions.

Service Tip

If skin is too dry or cold, wax may stick and will not come off properly. A tiny amount of lotion or oil may be used to pre-treat the skin. Conversely, too much product will prevent the wax from sticking. Make sure the room is warm so both the wax and client are at the right temperature. Check the wax consistency and machine temperature knob while setting up for services so adjustments can be made before starting a service.

Rubrics are used in education for organizing and interpreting data gathered from observations of student performance. It is a clearly developed scoring document used to differentiate between levels of development in a specific skill performance or behavior. Rubrics are provided in this supplement for use as either a self-assessment tool to aid the student in behavior development or as an educator assessment tool to determine competence. Space is provided to record steps needed for further growth and improvement.

Performance is evaluated according to the following scale:

1 Development Opportunity: There is little or no evidence of competency; assistance is needed; performance includes multiple errors.

2 Fundamental: There is beginning evidence of competency; task is completed alone; performance includes few errors.

3 Competent: There is detailed and consistent evidence of competency; task is completed alone; performance includes rare errors.

4 Strength: There is detailed evidence of highly creative, inventive, mature presence of competency.

Space is provided for comments to assist you in improving your performance and achieving a higher rating.

Leg Waxing with Soft Wax Assessment

PERFORMANCE ASSESSED	1	2	3	4	IMPROVEMENT PLAN
Preparation					
1. Completed standard pre-service procedure.					
2. Melted wax in heater for approximately 10 to 20 minutes.					
3. Placed clean sheet or single-use paper on waxing table.					
Procedure					
1. Cleansed area with mild astringent cleanser and dried.					
2. Applied light dusting of powder.					
3. Tested wax temperature and consistency.					
4. Used spatula or roller to spread a thin coat of warm wax evenly over skin surface in direction of hair growth.					
5. Began application 7" (17.5 cm) below the knee.					
6. Applied fabric strip in same direction of hair growth.					
7. Pressed gently but firmly, rubbing hand over surface of fabric 3 – 5 times.					
8. Held skin taut with one hand while removing wax in opposite direction of hair growth.					
9. Applied pressure to treated area for about 5 seconds.					
10. Repeated steps using fresh fabric strips.					

PERFORMANCE ASSESSED	1	2	3	4	IMPROVEMENT PLAN
11. Waxed below the knee working in three sections, across from one side to the other.					
12. Waxed top of knees above curve using same pattern.					
13. Had client turn over and repeated procedure on backs of legs.					
14. Removed any remaining wax residue.					
15. Applied an emollient or antiseptic lotion.					
16. Checked for and removed stray hairs.					
17. Removed gloves and washed hands.					
Post-Service					
1. Completed a post-wax consultation and discussed post-wax precautions.					
2. Completed standard post-service, cleanup, and disinfection procedure.					

Notes

_____

_____

_____

_____

_____

_____

_____

_____

_____

_____

_____

_____

_____

_____

18-5

PROCEDURE
18-6

Underarm Waxing with Hard Wax

IMPLEMENTS AND MATERIALS

The following list applies for all waxing procedures.

- Facial chair or treatment table
- Technician stool
- EPA-registered disinfectant
- Hand sanitizer
- Roll of single-use paper or paper towels
- Closed, covered waste container
- Cart
- Implement tray
- Containers for supplies
- Wax product
- Wax heater
- Wax remover
- Single-use applicators (large)
- Wax strips (for soft wax)
- Single-use gloves
- Sealable plastic bags for waste disposal
- Cotton pads and swabs
- Powder
- Mild skin cleanser
- Emollient or antiseptic lotion
- Brow brush
- Tweezers
- Small scissors
- Hand mirror
- Tongs (to retrieve clean supplies during a service)
- Surface cleaner (oil to remove wax from the equipment)
- Wax cleaning towels/supplies
- Table linens/towels
- Hair cap or headband for face waxing
- Towels for draping
- Client wrap for body waxing
- Wax release form and client chart
- Biohazard container, especially for underarm, bikini, and back waxing (the potential for blood spots from follicles is normal)

Preparation

- **Perform** 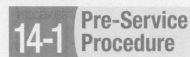 **14-1 Pre-Service Procedure** PAGE 16

- Melt the wax in the heater. Be sure the wax is not too hot.
- Complete the client consultation, release form, determine any contraindications, and determine what hair you need to remove.

Procedure

Because the hair under the arms grows in several different directions, it is important to first determine the number of different growth patterns and then to wax in sections following those patterns. Cut strips to the appropriate size if using soft wax. Divide the underarm area into multiple sections or as hair growth patterns allow. Follicles under the arm have fluids and spots of blood that come to the surface after hair removal, so apply a cold compress to calm the follicles after the hair is removed from the area.

1 Wearing gloves, cleanse the underarm area.

2 Apply a small amount of powder (or pre-wax product) to the area to dry the area and facilitate the adherence of wax. Have the client hold the skin taut next to the area to be waxed and place her hands where it does not interfere with the waxing pull. Hold the skin taut next to the edge of the wax strip where applying and removing the wax.

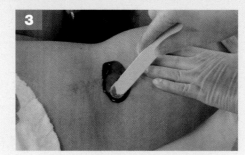

3 Apply wax to the first area, usually on the top or outer edge of the underarm. Leave a tab to grasp onto and check the consistency for removal.

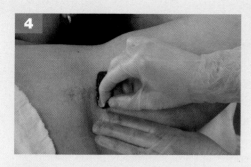

4 Remove wax: grasp the wax "handle" or strip and quickly pull. Hold and stretch the skin taut when removing the wax.

5 Apply pressure immediately after wax removal to ease any pain.

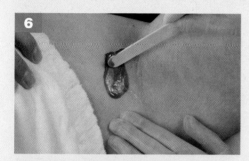

6 Repeat the procedure on the last growth area, or the center of the underarm. Remove any other stray hairs. Check-in with the client to make sure she is comfortable and can handle any tweezing. This is a sensitive area, so the faster the procedure, the better.

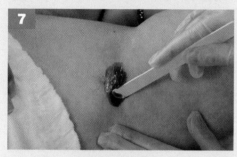

7 Repeat the procedure on the next growth area.

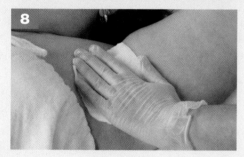

8 Apply a soothing after-wax lotion; cold compresses are also nice to soothe the skin.

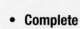
18-6

Post-Service

- **Complete** **14-2** **Post-Service Procedure** PAGE 22

- Complete a post-wax consultation and discuss post-wax precautions.

Rubrics are used in education for organizing and interpreting data gathered from observations of student performance. It is a clearly developed scoring document used to differentiate between levels of development in a specific skill performance or behavior. Rubrics are provided in this supplement for use as either a self-assessment tool to aid the student in behavior development or as an educator assessment tool to determine competence. Space is provided to record steps needed for further growth and improvement.

Performance is evaluated according to the following scale:

1   **Development Opportunity:** There is little or no evidence of competency; assistance is needed; performance includes multiple errors.

2   **Fundamental:** There is beginning evidence of competency; task is completed alone; performance includes few errors.

3   **Competent:** There is detailed and consistent evidence of competency; task is completed alone; performance includes rare errors.

4   **Strength:** There is detailed evidence of highly creative, inventive, mature presence of competency.

Space is provided for comments to assist you in improving your performance and achieving a higher rating.

Underarm Waxing with Hard Wax Assessment

PERFORMANCE ASSESSED	1	2	3	4	IMPROVEMENT PLAN
Preparation					
1. Completed standard pre-service procedure.					
2. Melted wax in heater for approximately 10 to 20 minutes.					
3. Washed and dried own hands.					
4. Put on disposable gloves.					
Procedure					
1. Cleansed and sanitized underarm area.					
2. Applied light dusting of powder (or pre-wax product).					
3. Tested wax temperature and consistency.					
4. Applied wax to first growth area.					
5. Held skin taut and grasped wax and quickly pulled to remove.					
6. Applied pressure immediately to ease discomfort.					
7. Repeated procedure on remaining growth areas.					
8. Removed stray hairs.					
9. Applied a soothing after-wax lotion or cold compresses.					
Post-Service					
1. Completed a post-wax consultation and discussed post-wax precautions.					
2. Completed standard post-service, cleanup, and disinfection procedures.					

Notes

Bikini Waxing with Hard Wax

IMPLEMENTS AND MATERIALS

Supplies will depend on the type of bikini waxing service to be performed (basic or Brazilian).

- Facial chair or treatment table
- Technician stool
- EPA-registered disinfectant
- Hand sanitizer
- Roll of single-use paper or paper towels
- Closed, covered waste container
- Cart
- Implement tray
- Containers for supplies
- Wax product
- Wax heater
- Wax remover
- Single-use applicators (large)
- Wax strips (for soft wax)
- Single-use gloves
- Sealable plastic bags for waste disposal
- Cotton pads and swabs
- Powder
- Mild skin cleanser
- Emollient or antiseptic lotion
- Brow brush
- Tweezers
- Small scissors
- Hand mirror
- Tongs (to retrieve clean supplies during a service)
- Surface cleaner (oil to remove wax from the equipment)
- Wax cleaning towels/supplies
- Table linens/towels
- Hair cap or headband for face waxing
- Towels for draping
- Client wrap for body waxing
- Wax release form and client chart
- Biohazard container, especially for underarm, bikini, and back waxing (the potential for blood spots from follicles is normal)
- Disposable underwear

Note: Soft wax with strips may be used in place of hard wax for the same procedure if performing an American or French bikini waxing (not a Brazilian wax).

Preparation

- **Perform 14-1 Pre-Service Procedure** PAGE 16

- Melt the wax in the heater. Be sure the wax is not too hot.
- Complete the client consultation, release form, and determine any contraindications.
- Place a clean sheet or sheet of paper on the waxing table for each new client.

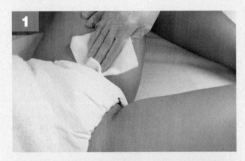

1 Wash hands and wear gloves. Drape the client. Tuck in a paper towel or wax strip along the edge of the client's bikini line. Cleanse the area.

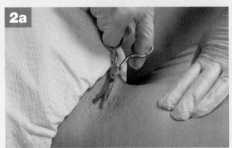

2a Trim the hair to ½" to ¾" (1.25 cm to 2 cm) in length if necessary.

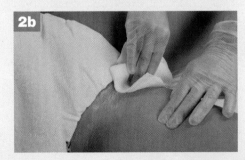

2b Apply a small amount of a pre-epilating product.

© Milady, a part of Cengage Learning. Photography by Dino Petrocelli.

3 Bend the client's knee with the leg facing out. This position assists in reaching the inner bikini area and stretches the skin tighter. Be confident in moving the client's body position around to reach the right angle for waxing, but make sure they are comfortable in the different positions.

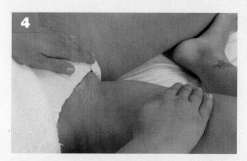

4 Have the client hold her skin taut next to the area being waxed. Show her where to place her hand and make sure that the hand is not in the way of the parallel pull used for removal.

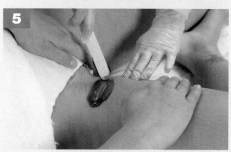

5 Apply wax to the first growth area, usually on the upper, outer edge of the bikini line. Extend the wax beyond the hair to make the pull tab and check wax consistency for removal.

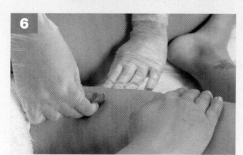

6 Remove the wax: hold the skin taut, grasp the wax "handle," and quickly pull. Pull back parallel to the skin.

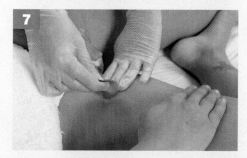

7 Apply pressure immediately to alleviate any discomfort.

8 Work in and down to the femoral ridge in sections. Do not wax over the curve of the femoral ridge (tendon).

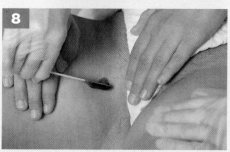

18-7

© Milady, a part of Cengage Learning. Photography by Dino Petrocelli.

18-7 Bikini Waxing with Hard Wax (continued)

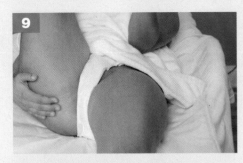

9 To wax the underside and the back side of the bikini area in separate sections have the client lift her leg toward her chest, grasping the ankle if possible. This position also holds the skin taut.

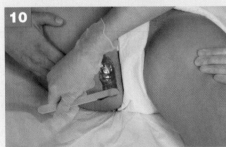

10 Apply the wax.

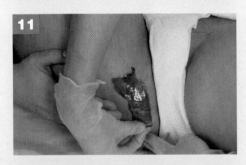

11 Remove it parallel to the body without lifting up while pulling.

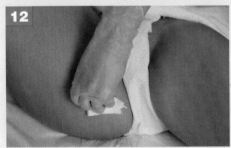

12 Apply a soothing after-wax lotion. (Cold compresses are also nice to soothe the skin.)

CAUTION!

Never go over the curve of the femoral ridge. Wax the top and bottom of the bikini area separately.

Post-Service

- **Complete** **14-2** PROCEDURE **Post-Service Procedure** PAGE 22
- Complete a post-wax consultation and discuss post-wax precautions.

Rubrics are used in education for organizing and interpreting data gathered from observations of student performance. It is a clearly developed scoring document used to differentiate between levels of development in a specific skill performance or behavior. Rubrics are provided in this supplement for use as either a self-assessment tool to aid the student in behavior development or as an educator assessment tool to determine competence. Space is provided to record steps needed for further growth and improvement.

Performance is evaluated according to the following scale:

1 **Development Opportunity:** There is little or no evidence of competency; assistance is needed; performance includes multiple errors.

2 **Fundamental:** There is beginning evidence of competency; task is completed alone; performance includes few errors.

3 **Competent:** There is detailed and consistent evidence of competency; task is completed alone; performance includes rare errors.

4 **Strength:** There is detailed evidence of highly creative, inventive, mature presence of competency.

Space is provided for comments to assist you in improving your performance and achieving a higher rating.

Bikini Waxing with Hard Wax Assessment

PERFORMANCE ASSESSED	1	2	3	4	IMPROVEMENT PLAN
Preparation					
1. Completed standard pre-service procedure.					
2. Melted wax in heater for approximately 10 to 20 minutes.					
3. Washed and dried own hands.					
4. Put on disposable gloves.					
Procedure					
1. Tucked paper towel or wax strip along edge of client's bikini line.					
2. Cleansed area with mild astringent cleanser and dried.					
3. Trimmed hair to ½" to ¾" (1.25 to 2 cm) in length if necessary.					
4. Applied light dusting of powder (or pre-epilating product).					
5. Bent client's knee with leg facing out.					
6. Made sure client was comfortable.					
7. Placed client's hands to hold skin taut.					
8. Applied wax to first growth area.					
9. Held skin taut.					
10. Grasped wax and quickly pulled back parallel to skin.					
11. Applied pressure to minimize discomfort.					
12. Worked in and down to femoral ridge in sections.					

PERFORMANCE ASSESSED	1	2	3	4	IMPROVEMENT PLAN
13. Waxed underside and back side of bikini area in separate sections.					
14. Had client lift leg toward chest.					
15. Applied wax and removed it without lifting.					
16. Applied a soothing after-wax lotion or cold compresses.					
17. Completed all requested services.					
Post-Service					
1. Completed a post-wax consultation and discussed post-wax precautions.					
2. Completed standard post-service, cleanup, and disinfection procedures.					

Notes

_____

_____

_____

_____

_____

_____

_____

_____

_____

_____

_____

_____

_____

_____

_____

Men's Waxing with Soft Wax

IMPLEMENTS AND MATERIALS

- Facial chair or treatment table
- Technician stool
- EPA-registered disinfectant
- Hand sanitizer
- Roll of single-use paper or paper towels
- Closed, covered waste container
- Cart
- Implement tray
- Containers for supplies
- Wax product
- Wax heater
- Wax remover
- Single-use applicators (large)
- Wax strips (for soft wax)
- Single-use gloves
- Sealable plastic bags for waste disposal
- Cotton pads and swabs
- Powder
- Mild skin cleanser
- Emollient or antiseptic lotion
- Brow brush
- Tweezers
- Small scissors
- Hand mirror
- Tongs
- Surface cleaner (oil to remove wax from the equipment)
- Wax cleaning towels/supplies
- Table linens/towels
- Hair cap or headband for face waxing
- Towels for draping
- Client wrap for body waxing
- Wax release form and client chart
- Biohazard container, especially for underarm, bikini, and back waxing

Due to the hair density, back waxing generally requires more wax strips. Strips fill up with hair quickly. Sometimes a partial wax will be requested and the time and price varies with the amount of waxing that is needed. Waxing of the back and neck is a common procedure for many men. First determine the number of different growth patterns, and then wax in sections following those patterns. Do not wax large strips of areas at one time—it's uncomfortable and traumatizes the follicles. Leg strip sections are generally too large. Cut the leg strips to three-quarters of the length. Save the unused leftover part of the strip for other body parts.

Preparation

- **Perform** 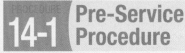 **PAGE 16**
- Melt the wax in the heater. Be sure the wax is not too hot.
- Complete the client consultation, release form, and determine any contraindications.
- Place a clean sheet or sheet of paper on the waxing table for each new client.

1 Have the client remove any uncomfortable clothing (belts) or give them a wrap to put on. Tuck a paper towel into the waist band to protect the clothing or wrap from wax. Have the client lay face down and start at the lower back area working up to the shoulders. Then have him sit up for the top of the shoulder area if necessary.

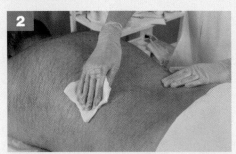

2 Cleanse the area to be waxed and trim hair as necessary. Brush excess hair onto a paper towel and discard before starting.

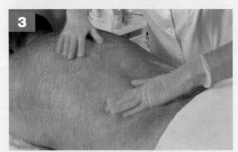

3 Apply a small amount of powder all over the area to be waxed. Check the hair growth pattern to decide on the pattern of removal before starting.

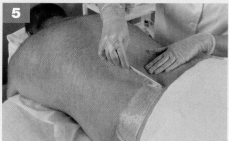

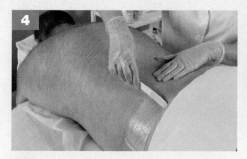

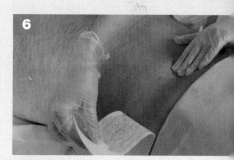

4 Apply wax to the first growth area. Start at the bottom of the lower back on the outside edge. Work in sections on one side of the body, working up towards the shoulders. Do the outside edge, then the center. Follow the hair growth and a set pattern.

5 Apply the strip. Do not use too big of a strip, as a large section is painful and the parallel removal is not as easy to control. Follow the directional changes. The client may need to turn onto their hip to wax the curved edge next to the bed, if the bed is in the way of the pull and follow through.

6 Grasp the strip, hold skin taut, and quickly pull parallel against the hair growth.

7 Apply pressure immediately after wax removal for at least 3 to 5 seconds to ease any pain. Apply cold compresses and soothing lotion as needed after completing a large section during the procedure.

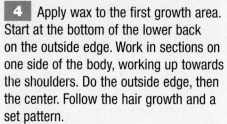

8 Repeat the procedure until all hair is removed, working up one side and then the other side of the body (this is more efficient to avoid changing sides during the waxing)

Service Tip

To wax a male client's shoulder and neck area, have him sit up and do the work from behind him.

Web Resources

www.dermatology.about.com

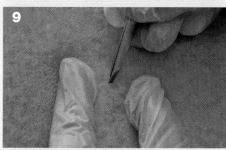

9 Remove any other stray hairs. Check-in with the client to make sure he is comfortable. It is a sensitive area, so the faster the procedure, the better.

10 Sit the client up to remove hair from the curve of the shoulder area. Blend the end of the waxed area to the front so there is not an abrupt line where the hairless area ends. Some trimming may be necessary here.

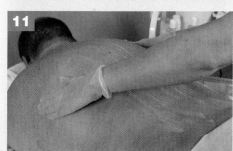

11 Apply a soothing after-wax lotion; large cold compresses (paper towels or cotton) are also used to soothe the skin. It is normal for hives and redness to appear after waxing such a large area of thick, coarse hair.

18-8

Post-Service

PROCEDURE
14-2 Post-Service Procedure

- **Complete** PAGE 22
- Complete a post-wax consultation and discuss post-wax precautions.

Rubrics are used in education for organizing and interpreting data gathered from observations of student performance. It is a clearly developed scoring document used to differentiate between levels of development in a specific skill performance or behavior. Rubrics are provided in this supplement for use as either a self-assessment tool to aid the student in behavior development or as an educator assessment tool to determine competence. Space is provided to record steps needed for further growth and improvement.

Performance is evaluated according to the following scale:

1 **Development Opportunity:** There is little or no evidence of competency; assistance is needed; performance includes multiple errors.

2 **Fundamental:** There is beginning evidence of competency; task is completed alone; performance includes few errors.

3 **Competent:** There is detailed and consistent evidence of competency; task is completed alone; performance includes rare errors.

4 **Strength:** There is detailed evidence of highly creative, inventive, mature presence of competency.

Space is provided for comments to assist you in improving your performance and achieving a higher rating

Men's Waxing with Soft Wax Assessment

PERFORMANCE ASSESSED	1	2	3	4	IMPROVEMENT PLAN
Preparation					
1. Completed standard pre-service procedure.					
2. Melted wax in heater for approximately 10 to 20 minutes.					
3. Determined number of different growth patterns.					
4. Cut leg strips to three-quarters of the normal length.					
5. Had client remove any uncomfortable clothing and lay face down.					
6. Washed and dried own hands.					
7. Put on disposable gloves.					
Procedure					
1. Cleansed area with mild astringent cleanser and dried.					
2. Applied light dusting of powder and checked pattern of hair growth for wax removal purposes.					
3. Tested wax temperature and consistency.					
4. Used metal or disposable spatula or roller to spread a thin coat of warm wax evenly over skin surface in direction of hair growth.					
5. Applied fabric strip in same direction of hair growth.					

PERFORMANCE ASSESSED	1	2	3	4	IMPROVEMENT PLAN
6. Pressed gently but firmly, running hand over surface of fabric 3 – 5 times.					
7. Held skin taut with one hand while removing wax and strip in opposite direction of hair growth.					
8. Applied pressure to strips for about 5 seconds.					
9. Pulled strip opposite to hair growth and parallel to skin.					
10. Applied pressure.					
11. Removed any stray hairs.					
12. Repeated steps using fresh fabric strips.					
13. Removed any remaining wax residue.					
14. Applied an emollient or antiseptic lotion, and cold compresses if needed.					
15. Completed all requested services.					
Post-Service					
1. Completed a post-wax consultation and discussed post-wax precautions.					
2. Completed standard post-service, cleanup, and disinfection procedures.					

Notes

_____

_____

_____

_____

_____

_____

_____

_____

_____

_____

18-8

20-1

Professional Makeup Application

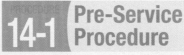

This is a basic makeup application. Your instructor may prefer a different method that is equally correct. Completing a makeup application includes the consultation, setup, application, and cleanup procedures. Some artists prefer to apply the makeup working from the top to the bottom of the face—eyes, cheeks, and then lips. There are pros and cons to every method. You will likely come up with your own prefered application procedure. If you miss a step, go back and perform it later if it does not complicate the application. The finished "painted" face is what is important, not how you get there. You may need to go back and change or add to your canvas once it is complete. It is, however, beneficial to develop a regular and efficient routine.

Preparation

- **Perform** **14-1** **Pre-Service Procedure** PAGE 16

- Start by setting out a few color selections: neutrals, cools, warms.

Procedure

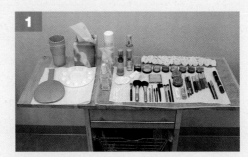

1 **Determine** the client's needs, and choose products and colors accordingly. Focus on your client's features and preferences. Discussing skin care or waxing is appropriate with a makeup client. Record these on the client chart. Ask the following questions:

- Do you wear contacts or have allergies?
- What look do you want?
- What makeup products do you normally wear?
- What are your typical clothing colors?
- What is the special occasion or event?

2 **Wash** your hands.

IMPLEMENTS AND MATERIALS

Skin Care Products
- Cleanser
- Toner
- Moisturizer (skin primer optional)
- Lip conditioner

Makeup
- Concealer
- Highlighter
- Contour color
- Foundation
- Powder
- Eye shadow
- Eyeliner
- Mascara
- Blush
- Lip liner
- Lipstick
- Lip gloss
- Other: bronzers, specialty items

Supplies
- Cape and draping supplies
- EPA-registered disinfectant
- Lined waste receptacle
- Tweezers
- Hair clip/headband
- Makeup brushes
- Pencil sharpener
- Mirror
- Lash comb
- Lash curler
- Hand towel
- Client charts

Single-use Items
- Spatulas
- Cotton (swabs and rounds)
- Mascara wands
- Sponges
- Tissues
- Applicators
- Paper towels

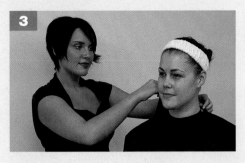

3 Drape the client and use a headband or hair clip to keep her hair out of her face.

4 Cleanser. After washing your hands, cleanse the face if the client is wearing makeup or if the skin is oily.

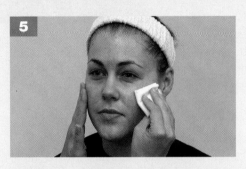

5 Freshener. Use a cotton pad to apply the freshener (or toner/witch hazel) to cleanse the skin.

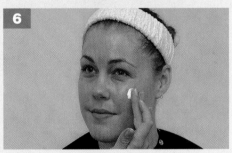

6 Moisturizer. Apply a small amount of moisturizer to prepare the skin for makeup. Apply a primer if applicable.

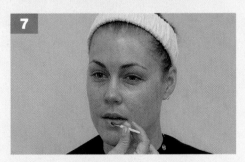

7 Lip conditioner. Use a spatula to remove the product from the container. Apply with a brush. To give it more time to soak in and moisturize, put on the lip conditioner when starting the makeup application.

Note: If lips are chapped, have clients rub off the dry skin with a wet wash cloth, esthetic wipes, or a lip scrub before starting the service. Tissue or paper towels are drying and leave lint on the lips so are not recommended for this.

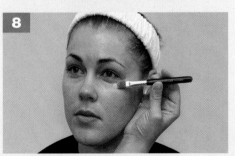

8 Concealer. Use a spatula to get the product out of the container. Choose a color one to two shades lighter than the foundation. You can apply this under or over the foundation beneath the eyes with a brush, sponge, or finger. Depending on the color, it can also be used as the highlighter (light) and to cover blemishes if it matches the skin tone. Apply using short strokes.

Note: Always use creams and liquids before applying powders, or they will not blend. If you are using a powder concealer or contour powder, apply these after the foundation.

20-1

© Milady, a part of Cengage Learning. Photography by Rob Werfel.

20-1 Professional Makeup Application (continued)

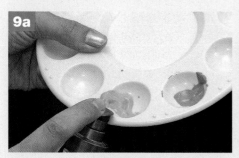

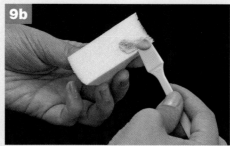

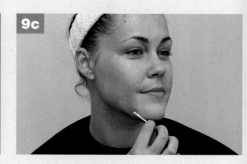

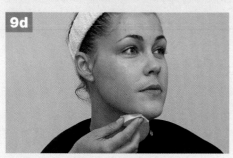

9 Foundation. First choose a few colors to match the right shade. Use a spatula to get the product out of the container, or put some on a clean sponge or in a small container. Apply to the jawline to match the skin color. Cover the skin using short strokes to even out the skin tone and cover imperfections without over-rubbing the skin. Blend along the jaw and edges of the face. Blend downward to blend with facial hair and up around the hairline so the product does not stick in the hairline. Pat gently around the eyes. Pressing, rather than rubbing, keeps the product on better.

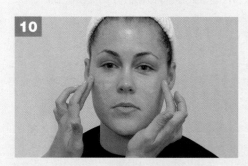

10 Highlighter. Use a spatula to get the product out of the container. Apply a white or light color to accentuate and bring out features along the brow bone, the temples, chin, or above the cheekbones. Blend with your brush, a sponge, or your finger.

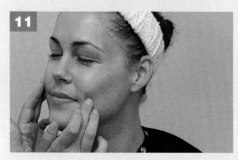

11 Contouring. Use a spatula to get the product out of the container. Using a small amount, apply a darker shade under the cheekbones and to other features you want to appear smaller. Blend well.

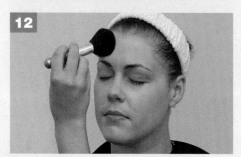

12 Powder. Pour a little powder on a tissue or tray to avoid cross-contamination. Apply to the brush and tap off excess powder onto the tissue (not the floor or table). Use a powder brush and sweep all over the face to set the foundation.

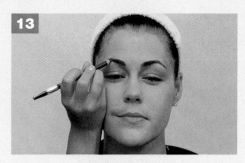

13 **Eyebrows.** Use a shade that is close to the hair color, or a shade the client likes. Apply color by using short strokes with a pencil or eye shadow with a brush. Smudge with a brush or a makeup sponge, going in the opposite direction of the hair growth to blend. Then smooth brows back into place with a brow brush.

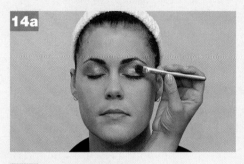

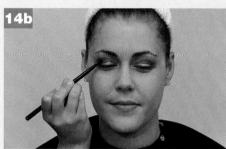

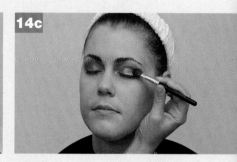

14a **Eye shadow.**

Light: Choose a light-base color and apply all over the eyelid, from the lash line up to the brow. Stop color at the outside corner of the eye up to the outside corner of the brow.

14b *Dark:* Apply a darker shade to the crease: partially on top of the crease and partially underneath the crease. First tap the excess powder off the brush. Apply the most color from the outside corner of the eye into the crease area above the inside of the iris.

14c This dark color covers three-quarters of the way above the outside part of the eye. Blend the color.

Optional: Apply the eyeliner before applying the dark shadow color.

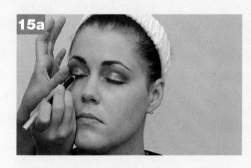

15a **Eyeliner**. Sharpen the liner before and after use.

Shadow as wet liner can also be used for liner and applied with a single-use or clean brush. Eye shadow can be applied as liner with a thin brush dipped in water. Dry shadow can also be applied with a thin, firm brush for a more natural look. Make sure the liner is not too rough or so dry that it drags on the eye. Liquid liners require applicators that are disposable or that can be disinfected.

Have the client shut her eyes when you apply the liner on top of the eyelids next to the lashes. Then have her look up and away as you apply the lower liner under the eyes. Apply the liner underneath the lower lashes.

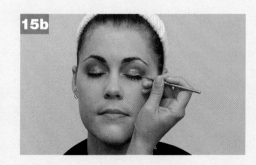

15b Bring the liner three-fourths of the way from the outside edge of the eye in towards the center of the eye, ending softly at the inside of the iris. Blend so that the color tapers off. Bringing the liner in closer to the nose can make the eyes appear closer together. Lining only the outside corner makes the eyes appear farther apart. Make sure the line does not abruptly stop. Blend the liner with a firm, small liner brush.

20-1

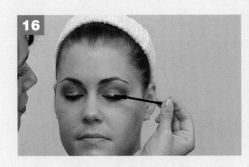

16 **Mascara.** Dip a single-use brush into the mascara. Move the wand from side-to-side from the base of the lashes out to the tips. Hold the wand at an angle (not pointing towards the eye) and apply more to the tips of the lashes.

Note: Some artists prefer to do the lower lashes first to avoid mascara touching the tops of the eye area when the client looks up for the lower application.

Bottom lashes: Wipe off the excess. Have the client put her chin down while looking up at the ceiling with her eyes to apply mascara to the bottom lashes. Comb and separate before the mascara dries.

Upper lashes: Have the client look down and focus on a fixed point to apply mascara to the upper lashes, brushing from the base to the tip. Comb with a lash comb before the product dries and before the client looks in a different direction to avoid smudging.

Use a cotton-tipped swab or small stiff brush with a little foundation or powder on it to fix or erase smudges.

Optional: Curl the lashes before applying mascara. Hold the curler on the base of the lashes without pulling and release the curler before moving it away from the lashes. Do not curl after mascara as lashes can be damaged and may fall out.

Optional: Apply false lashes following the mascara. Refer to Procedure 20–2, Applying Artificial Lashes, page 118.

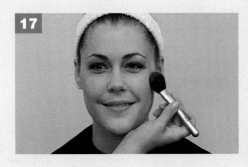

17 **Blush**. This can be done before the eyes. The blush color will depend on whether you choose a warm or cool color scheme. Tap off the excess powder on the brush. Apply blush just below the cheekbones, blending on top of the bones toward the top of the cheeks. Blend back and forth along the cheekbones. The color should stop below the temple and not be closer than two fingers away from the nose. It should not go lower than the nose, because this can "drag down the face." Blush should blend to the hairline, but not into it.

Do not apply too much blush on the apple of the cheek; this makes the face look fatter. A horizontal line makes the face appear wider, whereas a vertical line makes it look thinner. Following the cheekbones usually works best.

18 *Optional:* **Lip conditioner.** This step applies if lips are dry or you did not already apply lip moisturizer earlier. Use a spatula to get the product out of the container. Use a brush to apply. Put on a lip moisturizer when starting the makeup application so it can soak in and moisturize before you start applying the liner. If the lips have too much gloss or product, the liner will not go on or stick.

Optional: Some artists use a primer or foundation on the lips under the lip color to help keep it on, but these may be drying.

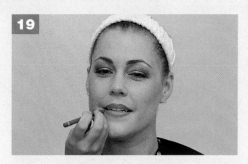

19 Lip liner. Sharpen the liner. Have the client smile and stretch her lips. With the lips pulled tight, the liner and lipstick brush glide on more smoothly. Line the outer edges of the lips first with small firm strokes; then fill in and use the liner as a lipstick. This keeps the lipstick and color on longer. Use a natural color for those clients who do not like liner. Lipstick will not last long without it.

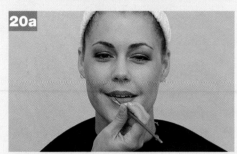

20a Lipstick. Use a spatula to get the product out of the container. Have the client select a color from among two or three choices. Apply the lipstick evenly with a lip brush. Rest your ring finger near the client's chin to steady your hand. Ask the client to relax her lips and part them slightly. Brush on the lip color. Then ask the client to smile slightly so that you can smooth the lip color into any small crevices.

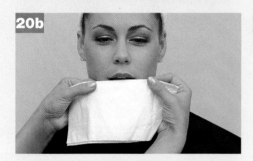

20b Blot the lips with tissue to remove excess product and set the lip color. Finish with gloss if desired.

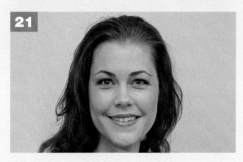

21 Show the client the finished application. Remove the cape and hair clips so you can see the finished look. Discuss the colors and any product needs she may have.

Post-Service

• **Complete** **14-2** **Post-Service Procedure** PAGE 22

• After the service is completed (and before the cleanup), fill out the client chart and make retail product suggestions and sales.

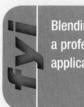

fyi

Blending is the key to a professional makeup application.

20-1

Rubrics are used in education for organizing and interpreting data gathered from observations of student performance. It is a clearly developed scoring document used to differentiate between levels of development in a specific skill performance or behavior. Rubrics are provided in this supplement for use as either a self-assessment tool to aid the student in behavior development or as an educator assessment tool to determine competence. Space is provided to record steps needed for further growth and improvement.

Performance is evaluated according to the following scale:

1 **Development Opportunity:** There is little or no evidence of competency; assistance is needed; performance includes multiple errors.

2 **Fundamental:** There is beginning evidence of competency; task is completed alone; performance includes few errors.

3 **Competent:** There is detailed and consistent evidence of competency; task is completed alone; performance includes rare errors.

4 **Strength:** There is detailed evidence of highly creative, inventive, mature presence of competency.

Space is provided for comments to assist you in improving your performance and achieving a higher rating.

Professional Makeup Application Assessment

PERFORMANCE ASSESSED	1	2	3	4	IMPROVEMENT PLAN
Preparation					
1. Completed standard pre-service procedure.					
2. Set out color selections.					
3. Determined client's needs. Cleansed own hands.					
4. Draped client and placed headband.					
Procedure					
1. Cleansed client's face.					
2. Applied freshener using cotton pad.					
3. Applied moisturizer.					
4. Applied lip conditioner with a brush.					
5. Applied concealer with sponge, brush, or finger.					
6. Chose the correct foundation shade.					
7. Applied to jawline to match the skin tone.					
8. Covered the skin to even out skin tone and cover imperfections.					
9. Blended along jaw and edges of face.					
10. Blended downward and then up and around hairline.					
11. Applied a white or light color to accentuate and bring out features along brow bone, temples, chin, or above cheekbones.					
12. Blended with brush, sponge or fingers.					

PERFORMANCE ASSESSED	1	2	3	4	IMPROVEMENT PLAN
13. Applied contour for shading and minimizing features.					
14. Applied powder to brush and tapped off excess.					
15. Used powder brush or puff to sweep downward all over face to set the foundation.					
16. Enhanced brows by using pencil or cake eye shadow with a brush.					
17. Smudged shadow with finger.					
18. Chose light-base eye shadow color and applied all over eyelid from lash line to brow.					
19. Applied a darker shade to the crease from the outside corner of the eye to the area above the inside of the iris.					
20. Sharpened liner before use.					
21. Applied liner on the upper lid from the outside of the eye toward the center of the eye as appropriate for how close-set the eyes are.					
22. Applied liner on the lower lid in a similar manner.					
23. Blended liner with a firm, small liner brush.					
24. Dipped disposable brush into mascara and wiped off excess.					
25. Applied mascara to top of lashes.					
26. Combed with lash comb before product dried.					
27. Applied mascara to bottom of lashes.					
28. Combed with lash comb before product dried.					
29. Applied blush to cheekbones as appropriate for face shape.					
30. Sharpened lip liner.					
31. Applied lip liner to outer edges of the lips.					
32. Filled in and used liner as a lipstick.					
33. Applied lipstick evenly with a lip brush.					
33. Blotted lips with tissue to remove excess product and set lip color.					
34. Showed the client the finished application.					
Post-Service					
1. Filled out the client chart and made product suggestions.					
2. Completed standard post-service, cleanup, and disinfection procedures.					

Applying Artificial Lashes

IMPLEMENTS AND MATERIALS

Supplies
- Disinfectant
- Headband or hair clip
- Tweezers
- Eyelash comb/brush
- Eyelash curler
- Hand mirror
- Small (manicure) scissors
- Adjustable light
- Adhesive tray or foil to put adhesive on
- Makeup cape
- Hand sanitizer
- Waste container

Products
- Artificial eyelashes
- Eyelid and eyelash cleanser
- Lash adhesive
- Eyelash adhesive remover
- Eye makeup remover

Single-use Items
- Cotton swabs
- Cotton pads
- Toothpick or hairpin
- Mascara wand
- Paper towels

Preparation

- **Perform** 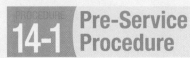 **Pre-Service Procedure** PAGE 16

- Discuss with the client the desired length of the lashes and the effect she hopes to achieve.
- Wash your hands.
- Place the client in the makeup chair with her head at a comfortable working height. The client's face should be well and evenly lit; avoid shining the light directly into the eyes. Work from behind or to the side of the client. Avoid working directly in front of the client whenever possible.
- Prepare for the makeup procedure, if applicable.
- If the client wears contact lenses, she must remove them before starting the procedure.
- If the client is only having artificial lashes applied and you have not already done so, remove mascara so that the lash adhesive will adhere properly. Work carefully and gently. Follow the manufacturer's instructions carefully.

Note: If the artificial lash application is in conjunction with a makeup application, complete the makeup either with or without applying mascara to the lashes, and then finish with the false lashes.

Procedure

1 Brush the client's eyelashes to make sure they are clean and free of foreign matter, such as mascara particles (unless this is part of a makeup application). If the client's lashes are straight, they can be curled with an eyelash curler before you apply the artificial lashes.

2 Carefully remove the eyelash band from the package. Tweezers work well for this.

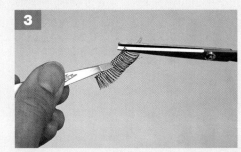

3 Start with the upper lash. If the band lash is too long to fit the curve of the upper eyelid, trim the outside edge. Hold this up to the eye to measure the length. Use your fingers to bend the lash into a horseshoe shape to make it more flexible so it fits the contour of the eyelid.

4 Feather straight band lashes to make uneven lengths on the end ("w" shapes) by nipping into it with the points of your scissors if desired. This creates a more natural look.

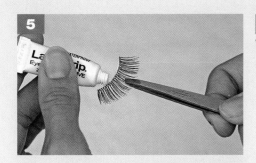

5 Apply a thin strip of lash adhesive to the base of the false lashes with a toothpick or hairpin and allow a few seconds for it to set.

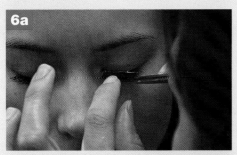

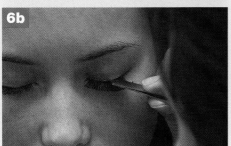

6 Apply the lashes by holding the ends with the fingers or tweezers. Make sure there is not an excess of glue and that the client can open their eyes once applied. Remove any excess glue and reposition the lashes as necessary.

For band lashes: Start with the shorter part of the lash and place it on the natural lashes at the inner corner of the eye, toward the nose. Position the rest of the artificial lash as close to the client's own lash as possible, not on the skin.

For individual lashes: Apply five or six lashes, evenly spacing each one across the lash line. Use longer lashes on the outer edges of the eye, medium length in the middle, and short on the inside by the nose. Cut lash lengths as needed.

Use the rounded end of a lash liner brush, the round side of a hairpin, or tweezers to press the lash on without adhering it to the glue. Be very careful and gentle when applying the lashes. Remove any excess glue and recomb or reposition lashes as necessary.

Note: Apply eyeliner before the lash is applied. An additional liquid liner may be used to finish the look if it does not affect the false lash adhesion. Adding a coat of clear mascara can help false lashes adhere to natural lashes.

7 *Optional:* Apply the lower lash, if desired. Lower lash application is optional; it tends to look more unnatural. Trim the lash as necessary, and apply adhesive in the same way you did for the upper lash. Place the lash on top or beneath the client's lower lash. Place the shorter lash toward the center of the eye and the longer lash toward the outer part.

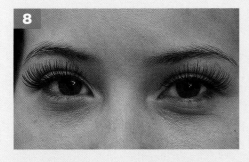

8 Check the finished application and make sure the client is comfortable with the lashes. Remind the client to take special care with artificial lashes when swimming, bathing, or cleansing the face. Water, oil, or cleansing products will loosen artificial lashes. Band lash applications last one day and are meant to be removed nightly. Individual lashes may last longer.

Post-Service

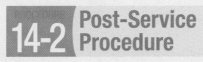

• **Complete** **14-2** **Post-Service Procedure** PAGE 22

Rubrics are used in education for organizing and interpreting data gathered from observations of student performance. It is a clearly developed scoring document used to differentiate between levels of development in a specific skill performance or behavior. Rubrics are provided in this supplement for use as either a self-assessment tool to aid the student in behavior development or as an educator assessment tool to determine competence. Space is provided to record steps needed for further growth and improvement.

Performance is evaluated according to the following scale:

1 **Development Opportunity:** There is little or no evidence of competency; assistance is needed; performance includes multiple errors.

2 **Fundamental:** There is beginning evidence of competency; task is completed alone; performance includes few errors.

3 **Competent:** There is detailed and consistent evidence of competency; task is completed alone; performance includes rare errors.

4 **Strength:** There is detailed evidence of highly creative, inventive, mature presence of competency.

Space is provided for comments to assist you in improving your performance and achieving a higher rating.

Applying Artificial Lashes Assessment

PERFORMANCE ASSESSED	1	2	3	4	IMPROVEMENT PLAN
Preparation					
1. Completed standard pre-service procedure.					
2. Cleansed own hands.					
3. Seated client in makeup chair.					
4. Had client remove contact lenses, if applicable.					
5. Removed mascara.					
Procedure					
1. Brushed client's eyelashes to remove foreign matter.					
2. Carefully removed eyelash band from package.					
3. Trimmed band from outside edge to fit the eyelid.					
4. Shaped lash band to the contour of the eyelid.					
5. Feathered lash ends to create a more natural look.					
6. Applied a thin strip of lash adhesive to the band with a toothpick or hairpin and allowed a few seconds to set.					
7. Applied band lashes by holding ends with fingers or tweezers and began with inner corner and worked outward.					
8. Placed band as close to natural lashes as possible.					

PERFORMANCE ASSESSED	1	2	3	4	IMPROVEMENT PLAN
9. For individual lashes, applied 5 or 6 lashes evenly spaced across the lash line using shorter ones in the inner corner and longer ones toward the outer corner.					
10. Optional: Applied the lower lash bands following the same procedure.					
11. Checked the finished application and made sure client was comfortable with the application.					
Post-Service					
Completed standard post-service, cleanup, and disinfection procedures.					

Notes

_____

_____

_____

_____

_____

_____

_____

_____

_____

_____

_____

_____

_____

_____

_____

_____

_____

Lash and Brow Tinting Procedure

IMPLEMENTS AND MATERIALS

Supplies
- EPA-registered disinfectant
- Headband
- Hand towels
- Plastic mixing cup
- Distilled water
- Small bowl of water
- Timer
- Brow comb or mascara wand
- Eyeliner brush
- Small scissors
- Lined waste container

Products
- Cleanser or eye makeup remover
- Witch hazel
- Petroleum jelly/occlusive cream
- Lash tint kits: black for lashes and brown for brows unless client requests otherwise

Single-use Items
- Cotton swabs (12)
- Round cotton pads (8)
- Protective paper sheaths (1 under each eye)
- Sealable sandwich bag (to discard waste in)

Preparation

- **Perform** **14-1** **Pre-Service Procedure** PAGE 16

Procedure

1 Wash hands.

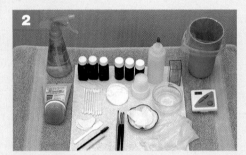

2 Gather and set out supplies.

3 Wet cotton pads and cotton swabs. Cut supply amounts in half if doing only one procedure on either the brows or lashes.

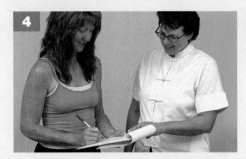

4 Conduct the client consultation, and have the client sign the release form.

© Milady, a part of Cengage Learning. Photography by Rob Werfel.

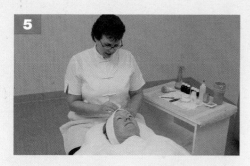

5   Drape the client with a headband and towel around the neck.

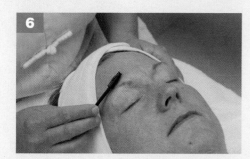

6   Wash your hands and cleanse the brow and/or lash area. All makeup must be removed and the area clean and dry before applying tint. Brush brows into place.

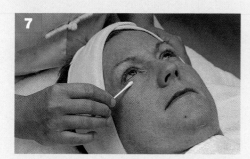

7   Apply protective cream with a cotton swab directly next to the area where you are tinting to protect the skin, covering the area where you do not want the tint. Do not touch the hairs with cream because this interferes with the color. Apply cream around the brow area. Apply under the eyelashes on the skin below the eye and above the lashes, just next to the lash line.

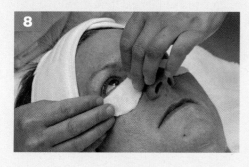

8   *For lash tinting:* Apply pads under the eyes and over the cream to keep tint from bleeding onto the skin. Use the paper sheaths in the tint kit, or you can make thin cotton pads from cotton rounds.

You may have to cut or adjust pad shapes to fit under the eyes. Pads should be under the lashes as close to the eye as possible without hoiding or interfering with the lower lashes.

To make cotton pads: Wet the pads and squeeze out excess water, tearing them so they are half as thick. Then fold in half to make half-moon shaped pads.

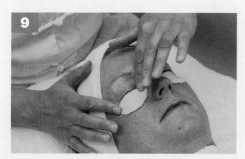

9   *For lash tinting:* Have the client close her eyes, and adjust the pad so it sits next to the eye—not bunched up too close to the eye. If the pad is too close or too wet, tint may wick into the eye and onto the skin.

Note: You can start with the lashes and do the brows while the lash tint is processing. Generally, tint can sit on the lashes longer than the brows if you are going for a natural brow-look.

20-3

20-3 Lash and Brow Tinting Procedure (continued)

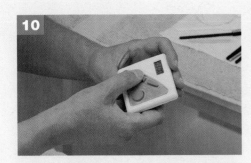

10 Set timer according to manufacturer's directions and have wet pads and cotton swabs ready to use for rinsing.

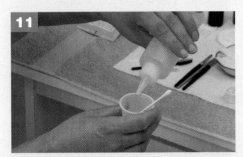

11 *For brows:* The tint can be diluted with water in a 1:1 ratio in a mixing cup to lighten the color.

Caution: Brows can absorb color quickly, so be ready to remove it right away to avoid excess color. Make sure you do not get your colors mixed up if using both brown (brows) and black (lashes).

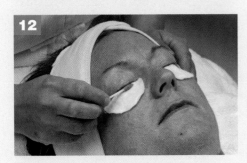

12 *Apply tint:* Dip cotton swab or brush applicator into tint (bottle #1), blot excess, apply and carefully saturate the lashes or brows. Brush on lashes from base to tip. Brush on brows from the inside out to the edge. A toothpick can be used to hold up the brow hair off of the skin while applying to avoid getting the product on the skin. Hold up different sections and work across the brow.

13 Leave on for 3 minutes or as directed. Some tint kits have only one bottle and combine the tint and developer into one application. Alter the procedure accordingly. Do not double-dip—use a new applicator each time to reapply.

CAUTION!

To avoid eye damage, do not let tint or water drip into the client's eyes. Have the client keep her eyes closed the whole time.

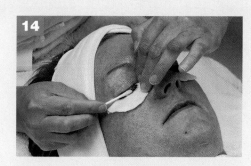

14 With a new applicator, carefully apply the developer (bottle #2 for some kits) for 1 minute or as directed.

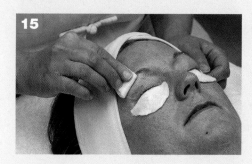

15 Rinse each area with water at least three times with wet cotton swabs and cotton pads without dripping water into the eyes.

Tip: Before rinsing, you can replace the under-eye shields if necessary (if color is bleeding through the pads to the skin). Make sure the tint does not touch the skin.

16 Ask the client if she feels any discomfort, and have her flush the eyes with water at the sink if necessary. It is common for the eyes to feel a little grainy after tinting, so rinsing is a good idea.

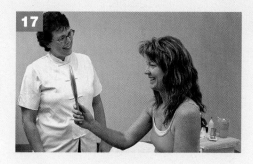

17 Show the application to the client.

Post-Service

- **Complete** **PROCEDURE** **14-2** **Post-Service Procedure** PAGE 22

- After the service is completed (and before the cleanup), fill out the client chart, and make any product suggestions and sales.

20-3

Rubrics are used in education for organizing and interpreting data gathered from observations of student performance. It is a clearly developed scoring document used to differentiate between levels of development in a specific skill performance or behavior. Rubrics are provided in this supplement for use as either a self-assessment tool to aid the student in behavior development or as an educator assessment tool to determine competence. Space is provided to record steps needed for further growth and improvement.

Performance is evaluated according to the following scale:

1 **Development Opportunity:** There is little or no evidence of competency; assistance is needed; performance includes multiple errors.

2 **Fundamental:** There is beginning evidence of competency; task is completed alone; performance includes few errors.

3 **Competent:** There is detailed and consistent evidence of competency; task is completed alone; performance includes rare errors.

4 **Strength:** There is detailed evidence of highly creative, inventive, mature presence of competency.

Space is provided for comments to assist you in improving your performance and achieving a higher rating.

Lash and Brow Tinting Procedure Assessment

PERFORMANCE ASSESSED	1	2	3	4	IMPROVEMENT PLAN
Preparation					
1. Completed standard pre-service procedure.					
2. Cleansed own hands.					
3. Gathered and set out supplies.					
4. Wet six cotton pads and swabs.					
5. Conducted consultation and had client sign release form.					
6. Seated client in makeup chair.					
7. Had client remove contact lenses, if applicable.					
8. Draped client with headband and towel around neck.					
Procedure					
1. Washed hands again and cleansed brow and/or lash area.					
2. Brushed brows into place.					
3. Applied protective cream with cotton swab directly next to area to be tinted to protect skin.					
4. Did not touch lash or brow hairs with protective cream.					
5. Applied pads under the eyes and over the cream to keep tint from bleeding onto skin.					
6. Prepared product for application.					
7. Dipped cotton swab or brush applicator into tint and blotted excess.					

PERFORMANCE ASSESSED	1	2	3	4	IMPROVEMENT PLAN
8. Carefully saturated lashes from base to tip.					
9. Carefully saturated brows from inside to outer edge.					
10. Set timer.					
11. Applied developer, if applicable, for the product choice.					
12. Had wet pads and cotton swabs ready to use for rinsing.					
13. After correct processing time, thoroughly rinsed tint from lashes					
14. Asked client how her eyes felt and had her flush at sink if necessary.					
15. Showed the finished look to client.					
Post-Service					
1. Filled out client chart and made product recommendations.					
2. Completed. standard post-service, cleanup, and disinfection procedures.					

Notes

_____

_____

_____

_____

_____

_____

_____

_____

_____

_____

_____

_____

_____

MILADY STANDARD

ADVANCED
ESTHETICS

Table of Contents

Excerpt from Milady Standard Esthetics Advanced: Step-by-Step Procedures ISBN-10: 113301349X
ISBN-13: 9781133013495. Order your copy today!

Thermotherapy for Clogged Pores

Implements and Materials

- Cleanser to remove makeup
- Stimulating massage product
- Antiseptic toner
- Standard facial lounge setup with linens and towels
- Gloves
- Disposable compresses, cloths, or sponges for removing product
- Water and bowl
- Steamer (optional)
- Treatment brush
- Enzyme exfoliant
- Cotton swabs or comedo extractor
- Serum to facilitate extraction
- Serum to soothe or calm the skin
- Hydrating serum
- Cool globes, high-frequency or sonophoresis
- Very warm wet towels
- Cool wet towels
- Sun protection

This procedure is designed to prepare and soften the impactions for extraction. Thermotherapy uses warmth and coolness to facilitate this process and calms the skin following the procedure.

Preparation

1 Set up the facial lounge with linens.

2 Prepare towels and cotton and gather supplies.

3 Decant or set up products.

Procedure

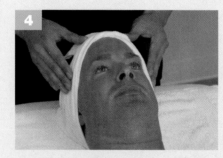

4 Prepare the client for treatment.

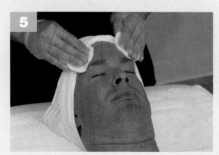

5 Cleanse. Moisten the skin using warm cotton compresses or sponges.

© Milady, a part of Cengage Learning. Photography by Rob Werfel.

Excerpt from Milady Standard Esthetics Advanced: Step-by-Step Procedures ISBN-10: 113301349X
ISBN-13: 9781133013495. Order your copy today!

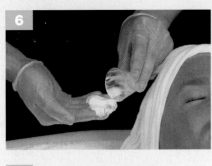

6 Apply a cleanser suitable to remove makeup with your gloved hands.

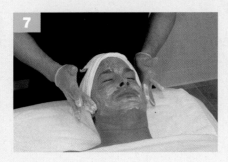

7 Massage the cleanser to loosen makeup.

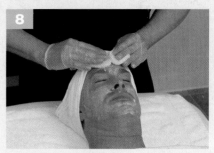

8 Remove the cleanser using warm cloth, sponges, or compresses.

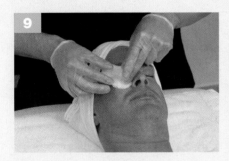

9 Place moistened eye pads on the eyes.

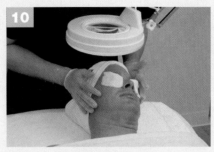

10 Examine the client's skin under a magnifying lamp. Observe for the level of sensitivity and skin response to cleansing. Confirm that the selected products and that the temperature changes planned will be appropriate.

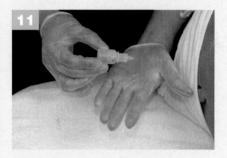

11 Apply a serum designed to loosen impactions. If you use warm steam, place the head of the steamer 18 to 20 inches (45 to 50 centimeters) from the client's face.

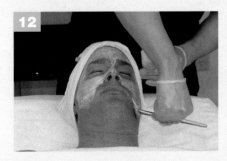

12 Use an enzyme exfoliant following the manufacturer's guidelines.

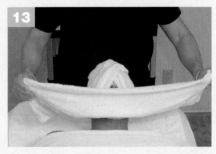

13 Wrap the face in two hot towels in a classical barber wrap. The towel should be very warm but comfortable. Place the second towel on top of the first.

14 Leave the towel on the skin for 8 to 10 minutes. If the towel cools too quickly, use steam to keep it warm or replace the top towel with a fresh one.

15 Remove top towel.

© Milady, a part of Cengage Learning. Photography by Rob Werfel.

Excerpt from Milady Standard Esthetics Advanced: Step-by-Step Procedures ISBN-10: 113301349X
ISBN-13: 9781133013495. Order your copy today!

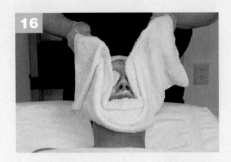

16 Use the lower towel to remove enzyme from the skin.

17 Before starting extraction, refresh your gloves if necessary. Apply a pre-extraction serum if desired. Follow the manufacturer's guidelines.

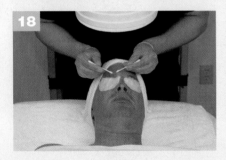

18 Use the cotton swab technique or a comedone extractor to perform extraction.

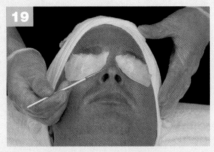

19 If the skin begins to welt, redden severely, or swell, stop extraction immediately. Limit the extraction to 5 to 10 minutes only, particularly during the first visit.

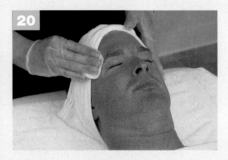

20 Wipe the skin with a soothing or antiseptic toner.

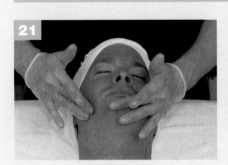

21 Apply soothing serum.

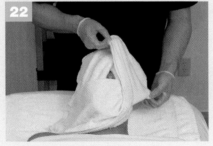

22 Apply cool wet towels, wrapping the face in a classical barber wrap. As an alternative, you can use cold globes over gauze, slowly stroking across the entire face, one area at a time.

23 Allow the skin to calm for about 10 minutes.

Excerpt from Milady Standard Esthetics Advanced: Step-by-Step Procedures ISBN-10: 113301349X
ISBN-13: 9781133013495. Order your copy today!

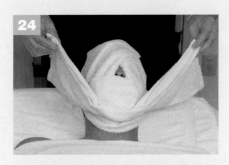

24 Remove towels.

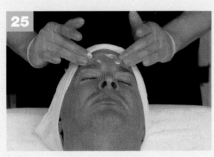

25 Apply a hydrating fluid and sunscreen.

Post-Procedure

26 Advise the client to treat any extracted area carefully and to avoid touching it. Advise the client not to apply makeup for at least two hours.

27 Remind the client to avoid the sun.

28 Determine whether the client is using appropriate home care products for his or her skin.

Clean-up and Disinfection

29 Perform clean-up and disinfection according to OSHA or state regulations.

30 Reset the room and prepare it for the next client.

31 Record detailed treatment information, observations, and product recommendations on the client service record card.

Excerpt from Milady Standard Esthetics Advanced: Step-by-Step Procedures ISBN-10: 113301349X
ISBN-13: 9781133013495. **Order your copy today!**

Notes